Functional Clinical Aesthetics™

by

Fortunata Calorigero
DBM, MScPhM, B.A., RCphT[cpd], LE et var.

© 2020 Fortunata Calorigero. All Rights Reserved.

Copyright in this work rests with the author. Please ensure that any reproduction or re-use is done in accordance with the relevant national copyright legislation.

Disclaimer.
This book has informational meaning and is not intended as medical advice.
The subject gives legal consent, in written form, to the sharing of personal informtion, medical history and all other data necessary to appropriately conduct the study, from the start to its completion.
The researcher/practitioner shall at all times act in accordance with the ascribed professional scope of practice and code of ethics.
It is expressly and clearly stated that no claims are/will be made upon complementary and alternative healthcare - in general - and related therapy(-ies), adopted during this case study – specifically –as intended to replace care from a qualified health provider or practitioner.
It is furthermore stated that, every and all claims related – but not limited to - to diagnose illness, make recommendations involving pharmaceutical drugs or surgery, or handle medical emergencies, are explicitly and implicitly rejected.
Be it stated that all and any tools, products, devices used during the course of this case study are not mentioned/adopted for advertising, nor promotional purposes.

© 2020 Fortunata Calorigero. All Rights Reserved.

Restrictions on Use. Materials available in this book are protected by copyright law and rest with the author. No reproduction or use, or storage in a retrieval system, or transmitted by any means are peritted without the written consent of the author.

Intellectual Property Copyright means all registered patents and not registered, copyrights, industrial designs and trademarks, trade names and all trade names, secret processes, trade secrets, engineering, design, process information and operation, inventions, developments, patents, trademarks, industrial designs and copyrights. All applications, technical data and other technical scientific information related to any process or method that is now owned or controlled by DBM. Fortunata Calorigero and that relates in any way to business, operations or activities of the Functional Clinical Aesthetics™ Model.

E-mail address: fortunata.calorigero@functionalclinicalaesthetics.com

Functional Clinical Aesthetics™ Model
Copyright Registration Number TXu 2-229-562
U.S. Trademark Application Serial No. 90005864

Credentials

Doctorate, Botanical Medicine
National University of Medical Sciences | Spain
Main Subjects:
Fundamentals of Botanical Medicine| Botanical Medicine Materia Medica| Herbology Principles, Practice, Ethics and Jurisprudence| Botany and Plant Identification| Diagnosis and Symptomology| Radiology| Applied Phytotherapeutics| Botanical Medicine Clinical Skills| Botanical Management of Musculo-skeletal Disorders| Practical Botanical Pharmacy| Clinical Nutrition.

Bachelor of Applied Science - BASc, Biotechnology - Laboratory Technology (in progress)
St. Petersburg College | FL, USA

Certificate, Biochemistry/The chemistry of Life
Kyoto University | KyotoUx Platform, Japan

Certificate in Clinical Dermatological & Cosmeceutical Compounding
American College of Apothecaries | TN, USA

Diploma Pharmacy Technology (RPT, CPhT)
Miami Dade College - Medical Campus | FL, USA

Skincare Specialist Program (LE)
World of Beauty Academy | FL, USA

Master's, Herbalism
S.A.C. - BTEC | UK

Diploma, Complementary Healthcare
Diploma, Anti-Ageing
Diploma, Medicinal Herbs
S.A.C. - BTEC | UK

Executive Master's in Management & Marketing for Pharmaceutical Industry
ALMA LABORIS Institute | Italy)
Main Subjects:
Pharmaceutical Management| Pharmaceutical Marketing| Procurement, Traceability and Logistics| Monitoring of the Processes and Quality Control of the Production| Human Resources Management in the Pharmaceutical Company | Management Control in the Pharmaceutical Field | Regulatory Affairs.

Bachelor's degree in Expert Languages for Business, Marketing and Management
University CATTOLICA DEL SACRO CUORE | Italy

et var.

Credentials

Author of the Functional Clinical Aesthetics™ Model

Inventor of the Oxypin™

CEO&Founder/Lecturer at Elixheal® Skincare
Manufacturer of clinical aesthetic products for professional use.

Educator/Consultant at Academia de Estética Clínica Avanzada
Medicina Funcional Aplicada a la Estética Clínica
Principios de Ciencia Cosmética

CEO/Lecturer at MESOTECHUSA
Italian manufacturer of Medical Devices & Products for aesthetic medicine.

RCPht at Jackson Memorial Hospital
Non-sterile Compounding and misc.

CPht at Universal Arts Compounding Pharmacy
Intern non-sterile Compounding.

International Business Development Manager at MESOTECH Italy
Italian manufacturer of Medical Devices & Products for aesthetic medicine.

Proud Member of:

SCC - FL Chapter
(Society of Cosmetic Chemists)

ORCID
(Open Researcher and Contributor ID)

NWU
(National Writers Union)

OWIT
(Organization of Women in International Trade)

NNA
(National Notary Association)

Table of Contents

INTRODUCTION... viii

Part I: The Initial Assessment

CHAPTER ONE
Gathering the Information... 10

CHAPTER TWO
Information vs Knowledge, connecting the dots................ 14

Part II: The FCA™ Model

CHAPTER THREE
From the Aesthetic Condition to the Root Cause................ 18

CHAPTER FOUR
A Customized Therapeutic Program...26

CHAPTER FIVE
Comparative Findings... 44

CONCLUSION.. 117

BIBLIOGRAPHY.. 119

INTRODUCTION

The Functional Clinical Aesthetics™ Model is a pioneering approach based on applications of CAM doctrines to conventional methods of wellness and beauty care.

Resorting to Complementary and Alternative Medicine, with a particular focus on Functional Medicine and Phytomedicine's know-how, the Functional Clinical Aesthetics™ Model, or FCA™ Model, underlines causes of dysfunctions/imbalances through a deduction-driven approach, for a broader understanding of the nature of the aesthetic imperfection(s) and aims at developing a personalized-unique therapeutic program to treat and enhance, on a first standpoint, the overall health status with the ultimate goal of betterment of the aesthetic conditions from within.

Although this avantgarde approach might be often associated with disciplines that range from integrative dermatology to holistic beauty therapies, it is important to understand three main points:

1. The Functional Clinical Aesthetics™ Model encompasses all the "concerns" that can be considered aesthetic flaws/conditions (hair, nails, localized adiposity, etc.), not only aesthetic imperfections that are related to the skin.

2. The FCA™ Model utilizes a systematic approach that blends the know-how of a conventional aesthetic practitioner with CAM applications to analyze and assess beauty concerns from the root cause and therefore develop a personalized therapeutic program, unique to the needs of the customer in care.

3. The personalized therapeutic program consists of a custom protocol with multifunctional organic preparations. Natural ingredients only. Thoroughly selected and backed by evidence-based science from thousands of scientific papers and clinically effective results.

Cruelty Free, Parabens Free, Fragrance Free, Dyes Free, Alcohol Free.

Part I: The Initial Assessment

CHAPTER ONE
Gathering the Information

CASE IDENTIFIER

"FunctionalClinicalAestheticsModel"

SUBJECT HEALTH HISTORY

Details:

Born 02/22/1986

Age 34

Ethnicity: Caucasian – Fitzpatrick type III
Non-smoker, no drugs, no medications, social drinker.

Origin of the scar: injury from outdoor activity in 2014. Small wound's depth approx. 7mm.

After irrigation, the wound was treated with a liquid compound of Sodium DNA 3% and Tocopherol 0.5%, applied topically, with a dropper, twice a day, for 7 days (ref. to photo 1 and 2).

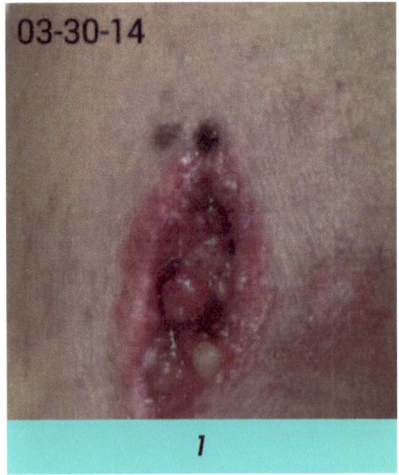
1

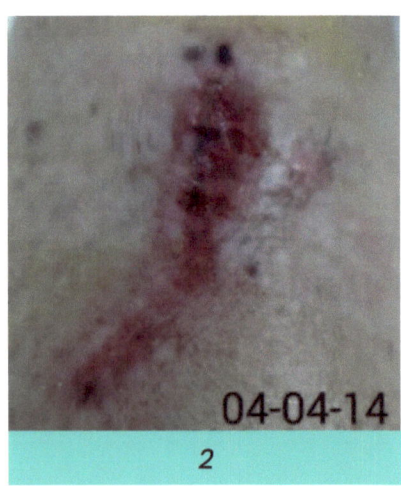
2

A sterile butterfly closure was used to close the wound.

No more treatments have been received on the area ever since.

2020: the subject currently presents a normotrophic skin scar and light dyschromia on left lower leg, front view, proximal to the extensor retinaculum muscle.

Scar size is approx. L 2cm x W 1cm. (ref. to photo 3 and 4).

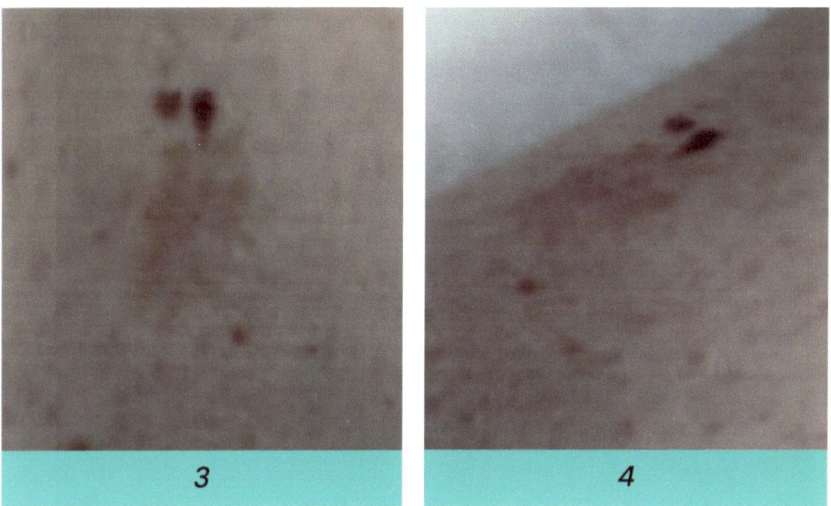

3   4

Parallelly to the main topic in object, a concurrent trial will be run on the subject, solely using the ad hoc compounds formulated accordingly with the results from the assessment techniques and devices used for health evaluation's purposes.

Area: Hands.

Condition: Glycation.

(ref. to photo 5 and 6).

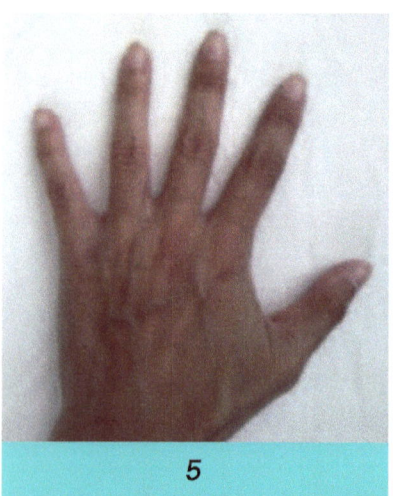

5

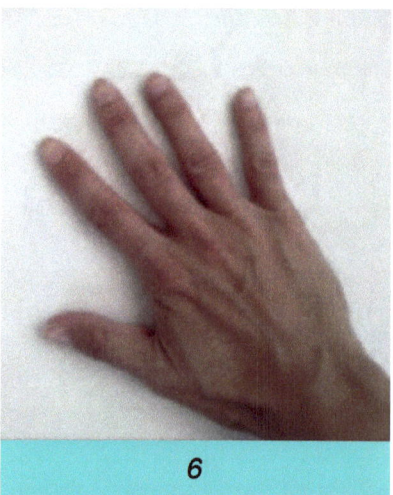

6

EXPECTED RESULTS

Reduced appearance of preexisting scarred tissue and dyschromia. Overall improvement of health conditions reflected on glycated skin area in analysis.

POSSIBLE OBSTACLES

Subject's adherence to the protocols of the therapy.
Subject decides to stop the therapy due to the perception that the benefits of the care do not outweigh the discomforts.

Unforeseen side effects/interactions.

CHAPTER TWO
Information vs Knowledge, connecting the dots

This case study starts with a definite path to be followed. Analyze the overall aesthetic flaw/condition through a set of conventional techniques and tests. From there, the focus passes on the results obtained from the CAM techniques and tools used for a comprehensive health assessment. Each condition detected is indexed accordingly (A, B, C, D, E...) and to each is associated a "liaison" on a physiological level (x, xy, xx, yy, yx.....), so to determine the possible root cause(s) in connection with the imbalances of the core processes. Once established their connection, a personalized therapeutic program is developed. The primary purpose is to trigger the activities of the systemic functions and to lead the healing process towards the aesthetic flaws/conditions being the main object of attention.

It is considered "the functional medicine operating system", as shown in figure 1 (Bland, 2015).

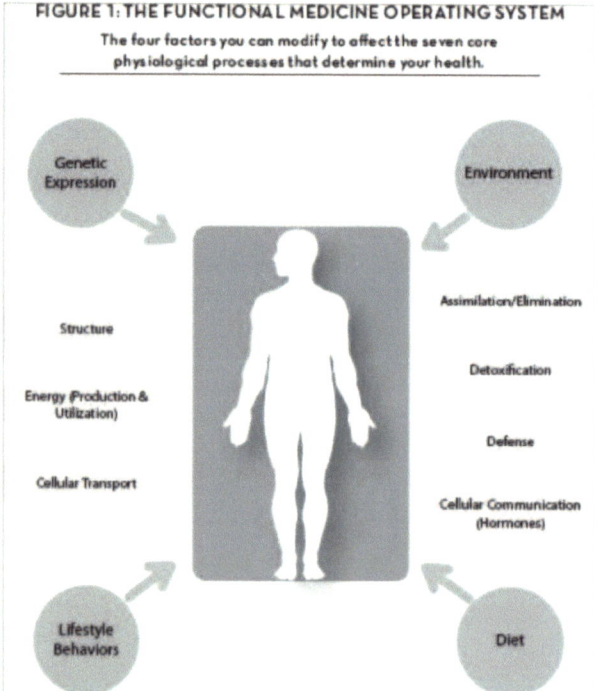

Figure 1

Once the information is available and the "dots" are connected, a new level of knowledge is achieved, which allows to develop a personalized therapeutic program to trigger the healing process.

The healing process will be effective both on the overall aesthetic flaw condition AND on a systemic level towards the core processes and their dysfunctions.

The FCA™ Model can be applied to any type of aesthetic imperfection.

Follows a practical application of the model in order to establish its validity.

Part II: The FCA™ Model

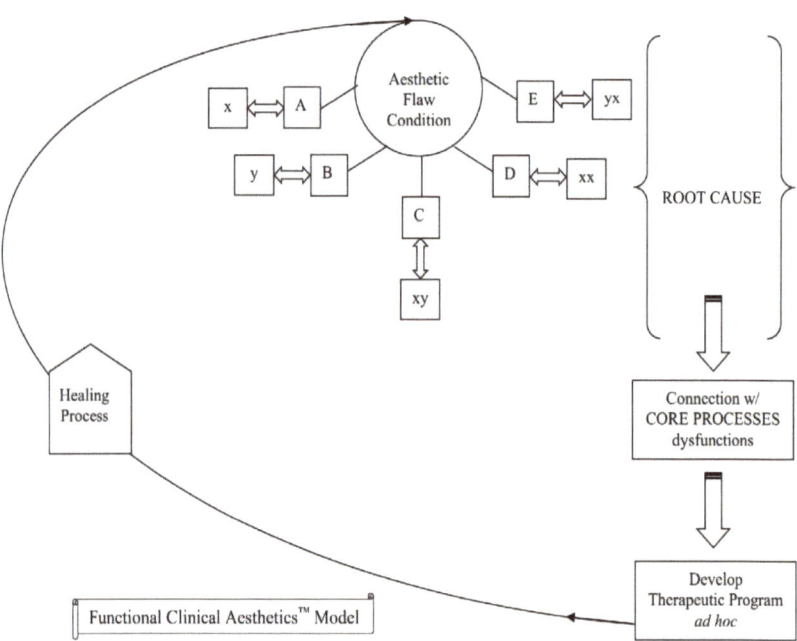

CHAPTER THREE
From the Aesthetic Condition to the Root Cause

Comprehensive Health Assessment

Test results from 05/29/20 and 06/03/2020

In this case study are only considered object of interest the results showing values between:

⋄ 5-6, expressing "decompensation of adaptation mechanisms; pathological state", as far as the NLS analysis is concerned.

⋄ Mildly abnormal (-/+) to severely abnormal (-/+), as far as the Magnetic Resonance Quantum Analysis is concerned.

The main object of interest will be the integumentary system and related physiological processes that affect its conditions.

Overall, the subject shows high stress levels, very close to a nervous breakdown, due to negative life events taking place. These stress levels reflect on:

⋄ Poor nutrition and sleep – the subject weight/height, during this study, is 95lbs/"5.01". BMI 19.1, borderline underweight. Waist circumference is approx. 60cm/23in. Depleted.

⋄ Compromised functions of cerebrovascular system, resulting in fatigue, lack of will and loss of focus.

⋄ Compromised functions of the lymphatic system, concurrently affecting thyroid gland activity, gastrointestinal functions on the level of absorption's coefficient, and kidneys for of fluid balance and detox.

⋄ Degeneration of skeletal system, highlighting vertebrae and long bones, co-related with circulatory disfunctions throughout the body, with specific focus on the arteries of head and neck, and brain with specific focus on the arteries of cerebrum, left hemisphere.

⋄ Cardiovascular activities are as well mildly deficient, resulting in a reduction of respiratory capacity.

⋄ Nervous system disfunctions impose on nerves of maxilla and mandibula, neck and stomach.

The skin appearance replicates the mentioned imbalances, in terms of:

- Lack of elasticity
- Increase of TEWL
- Glycation
- Mild exfoliating activity on arms and thighs.

Aesthetic Conditions

From an external observation the skin shows signs of high TEWL and lack of elasticity. Glycation is primarily evident on hands. Degenerative tendency to skin thinning.

Index

A. Increased level of Free Radicals
B. Mildly low level of Skin Collagen
C. Moderately high level of Skin Moisture
D. Moderately high Melanin level
E. Oily Skin level Mildly high
F. Mildly high traces of RBC on skin

Connections on Physiological Level

A-x. ROS (Reactive Oxygen Species). Damage body proteins, DNA and cells.
Metabolic processes produce free radicals for conversion of glucose into energy.
Phagocytes use free radicals to kill bacteria.
Due to hypoxia, mitochondria produce caustic oxidation substances. When these substances' levels are too high the system can't manage them, which results in DNA damage and therefore damage of the genetic message and genome. The mitochondria experience the corrosive effect of oxygen from free radicals. UV rays trigger the inflammatory process

in the skin, resulting in macrophages' production of high levels of O_2^-, superoxide anion, and T cells' production of ClO^- to kill harmful microbes (Lobo, Patil, Phatak, Chandra, 2010).

B-y. Collagen Type I and III is found in skin. The ECM - Extra Cellular Matrix – in the dermis contains generally high levels of collagen, resulting in tissue elasticity and firmness.
Fibroblasts in the dermis are the cells responsible for the integrity of the ECM to form collagen and elastin fibers. The degradation of the ECM occurs as well via release of metal-binding enzymes MMPs – Metalloproteinases – due to inflammatory process from Oxidative Stress response. Neutrophils' elastases activity and other proteases inactivates TIMPs, so inducing MMPs' expression (Pillai, Oresajo and Hayward, 2004).

C-xx. It is assumed that excessive skin moisture induces the depletion of the skin barrier, loss of water from the skin is known as TEWL – TransEpidermal Water Loss. There's no exact evidence related to the causes of its occurrence, though several mechanisms play a role in the process.

The temperature regulating activity from the sweat glands corresponds to the 4/5 of water loss, notwithstanding, the main cause is associated to the alterations of the lipidic layer of the barrier zone, composed by cholesterol and keratin, located between the *Stratum Spinosum* and the *Stratum Corneum* (Hibbott, 1963). Overhydration of the skin will result in the swelling of the corneocytes in the SC, leading to the expansion of the intercellular space and therefore "porosity" in the barrier zone, which will be vulnerable to the reduction of NMF – Natural Moisturizing Factor – and increase of TEWL.

Surfactants have as well an altering role on the lipid barrier in the and on the disrupture of the lamellar structure in the SC. A peripheral role might be considered in accordance with the Na^+/H_2O fluid imbalance due to the kidneys' inability to regulate the adequate H_2O intake.

D-xy. Melanosomes are the pigment-granules of melanocytes, or dendritic cells, containing melanin. The melanosomes are transferred from the melanocytes to keratinocytes in the SC to protect the cell nucleus from ultraviolet (UV) light. The process is activated by UV radiations, which trigger the production of nitric oxide, mediator of cellular metabolism, brought about by the enzyme *tyrosinase*. The inflammatory response to UV rays takes place in the "living" layers of the skin, causing the release of Interleukin-1, IL-1, from the SC, therefore stimulating the intercellular adhesion molecule-1, ICAM-1, expression of keratinocytes and alpha-melanocyte-stimulating hormone a-MSH). The sex hormone$a$-MSH induces the melanocytes production of more melanin for protection of skin from further UV damage (Pillai, Oresajo and Hayward, 2004). Adrenocorticotrophic hormone and pituitary gland can stimulate melanogenesis as well.

E-yy. Affected by hormones, sebaceous glands produce a fatty substance, sebum, consisting of free fatty acids, triglycerides, waxes, cholesterols, squalene, etc. Sebum forms a thin film over the surface of the skin to inhibit the growth of bacteria. When a certain amount of sebum and keratin occlude the skin pores, blackhead will manifest. Common skin disorders are the results of an inflammatory response of the sebaceous glands, resulting in an overproduction of sebum.

F-yx. The dermis layer of the skin is richly vascularized, and it extends into capillary loops up to the junction with the epidermis. Inflammation reaction from skin injury or other chemical or physical stimuli, will cause a dilation of the capillaries, resulting in skin reddening. Telangiectasia is a common condition related to the visibility on the skin surface of dilated capillaries with a tendency to break due to low levels of elasticity of vessels' walls. Vasoconstriction in the dermis may also occur in stressful situations.

Root Cause - CAM and Functional Medicine Interoperability Levels

Always remember that cells have memory.

From this point, the next step is to detect the root cause, restore the balance of the processes and the proper functions of the system.
Upon this premise Hering's Law of Cure comes in handy. This is based on the general concept that ailments/conditions "*originate*" by breaking down natural defenses according to the way one eats, drinks, thinks and lives. The healing process starts from within outward, from the inner parts of the body – mental and emotional levels and the organs – to the outer parts, such as skin and extremities.
A valid example can be given if considering how the accumulations of toxins from inside the body are expelled toward the outside throughout the skin.

Brain>Heart>Endocrine>Liver>Lung>Kidney>Bone>Muscle>Skin

From a functional medicine perspective, on the other hand, the following factors are to be accounted for, taking place in the tough central phase of the Covid-19 pandemic:

Environment: from February to April 2019 the subject has been remodeling house with her partner. The relationship break-up in May 2019 left the subject to cope alone with the unfinished house, the remodeling stopped. The subject has been highly exposed to dusts and heavy metals from construction materials from unfinished bathroom, no interior doors, open walls, no floors, no kitchen, and so on.

Diet: Poor diet lacking disciplined meals. Not enough protein intake. Not drinking enough water. High consumption of sugars. Subject doesn't take supplements or pharmaceuticals. No use of drugs nor alcohol.

Lifestyle: The subject started a new relationship in January 2018, in June 2018 moved from South of FL to the Gulf Coast of FL, planning to build a family with her companion. Bought a house and started remodeling. In the meanwhile, was enrolled in college, A.S. biotechnology, managing her own company and financially involved in an investment property. High stress levels created turmoil in the relationship and when Covid-19

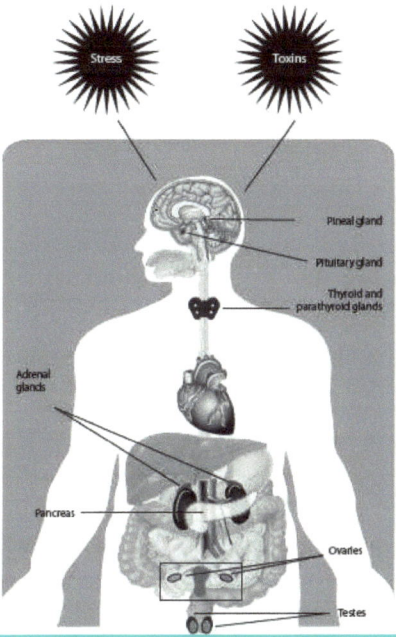

Figure 2 - The Hormonal Communication Process. Bland, J. S. (2014).

hit, in February 2019, all started to go downhill.
Due to Covid-19 subject experienced business' shut down causing a significant financial loss; investment property turned out to be a $30K loss; stress from house remodeling and college influenced badly the relationship stress levels resulting in a break up. No time dedicated to outdoor activities nor exercise or relaxation techniques.

Genetic Expression: No genetic disposition towards disease or specific conditions in relation to the mentioned indexes object of interest. Born and raised in the South of Italy. Family and ancestry deeply rooted culture and traditional background. Moved to the South of FL in 2013 and from there to the Gulf Coast in 2018. The genetic expression has undergone changes, creating a shift in the function of the core processes, which altered the symbiosis with the new environment. On the long term the self-regulating mechanism of adaptation failed so affecting the subject's health.

The information collected show that the subject has been in "survival mode" for the last 5 months up to July 2019. Structure and Cellular Communication (Fig.2) are identified to be at the root cause of the imbalance. The ongoing fight-or-flight response mechanism in action produces a resistance to the message, generating a GAS – General Adaptation Syndrome. This last reflects on the inability of the endocrine system to resist physiological stress.

The thyroid gland shows in thyroglobulin dysfunctions. Hormones of the adrenal medulla, epinephrine and norepinephrine, regulated by the hypothalamus (Sympathetic Nervous System) and parathyroid gland's PTH concur to lowering the rate of cellular respiration, and gastric peristalsis. In addition, PTH affects metabolism of calcium and phosphorus – $Ca(PO_4)^2$ – resulting in long bone healing deficiency and bone degeneration (osteoclasts functions, increase of bone hyperplasia, reduction of bone mineral density). Among the end products of this imbalance are inflammatory bowel conditions connected to the CNS by action of Vagus Nerve generating low impulses to the pylorus sphincter, so causing dysfunction of gastric peristalsis and absorption, small intestine peristalsis, colonic absorption, Intestinal bacteria, intraluminal pressure. From the small intestine Ca^+, P, and Vit. D are needed for the absorption of Vit. A and Vit. C, necessary for the process of bone matrix formation - ossification and calcification. The imbalance extends to ovaries and other bystanders: cardiovascular system, digestive system, bones, skin, muscles, and kidneys. Myocardial blood demand and oxygen consumption mildly high, assumes an issue with contracting proteins, myosin and actin, causing loss of cardiac action potential – connected dysfunction with sympathetic nerves in the medulla therefore reducing the stretching of the cardiac muscle so lowering the ANP levels. This last, together with Aldosterone by Adrenal cortex increases the reabsorption of Na^+ equals excessive excretion of K^+ and H^+ to prevent excessive accumulation so to avoid acidic pH and promote the reabsorption od Cl^- and HCO_3^- in the blood, retaining H_2O so increasing BP. Aldosterone as well affects Blood Volume levels reflecting in mild hypoxia, possible to result in cellular death and memory loss. The skeletal system analysis shows a debilitation of the vertebral column, directly affecting the spinal cord in transmitting impulses to and from the brain, and therefore the adequate activity of the nervous system and body as a whole. The spinal nerves C5-C7, T1-T2, T4-T12, L1-L5, and by extension the respective nerve plexuses, contribute to the dysfunction whose end destinations are primarily skin and muscles.

CHAPTER FOUR
A Customized Therapeutic Program

PROCEDURE (PROTOCOL, SESSIONS, CHANGES)

Approach:

Comprehensive acknowledgement of the subject's history and data on hand. Assessment of the subject's current condition and its persistence. Identification of possible root cause(s) triggering the subject's organism dysfunctions. Practical applications of theoretical studies from a number of CAM doctrines in order to develop an "ad hoc" therapeutic program for the subject.

A non-stop therapy of impact will be conducted.

Note: *Some of the values may result altered due to the subject being on menstrual cycle from 06/22 to 06/28.*

Devices, tools and products:

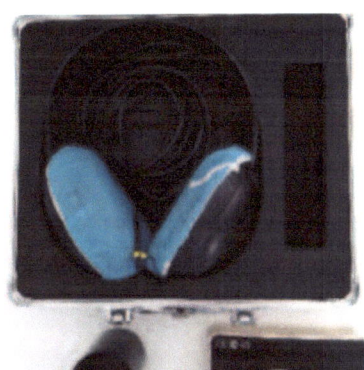

18D Metatron NLS body scan

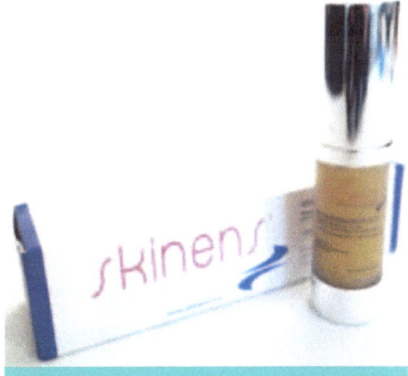

Multiactive viscoelastic creamigel

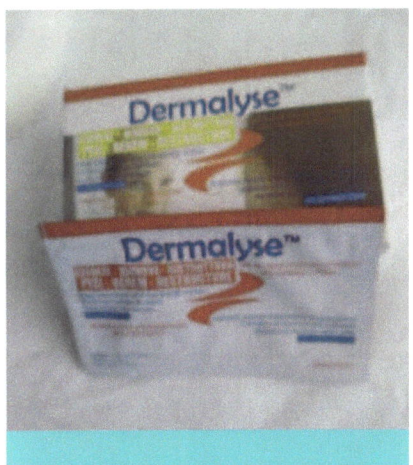

Mechano-chemical peeling gel

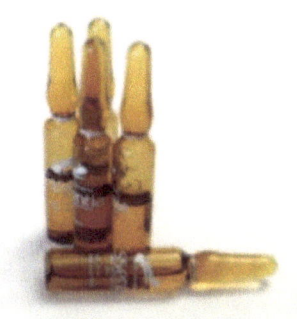

Mesocomplex Actives formulation

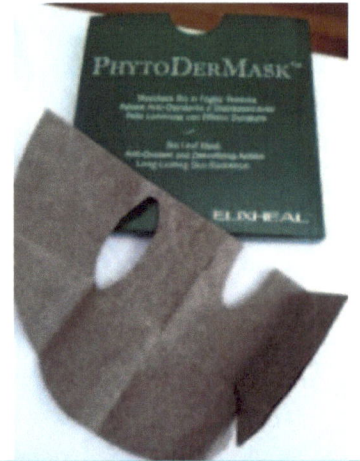
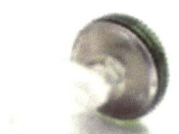

Woven-leaf Herbal patch (Camelia Sinensis Leaf, Mentha Piperita Leaf)

Micropin head 198 pins, size 0.5mm

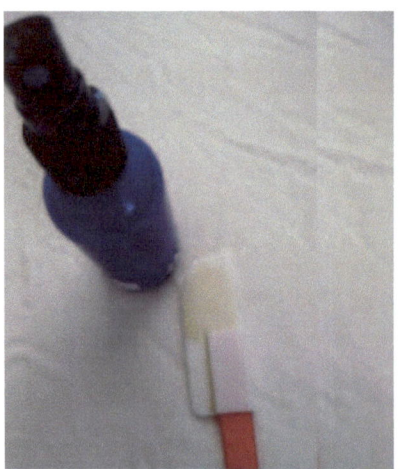
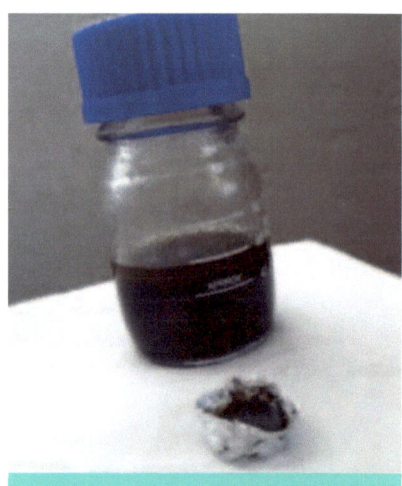

Topical lotion formulated ad hoc

Oral liquid preparation formulated ad hoc

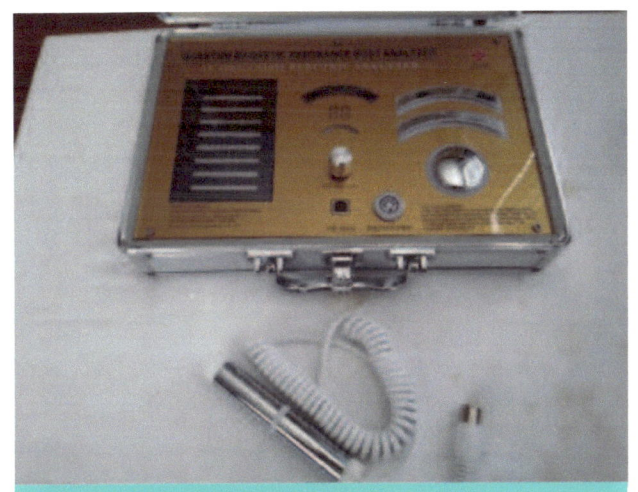

Magnetic Resonance Quantum Analyzer WF-QA46 (Biochemical Analysis System)

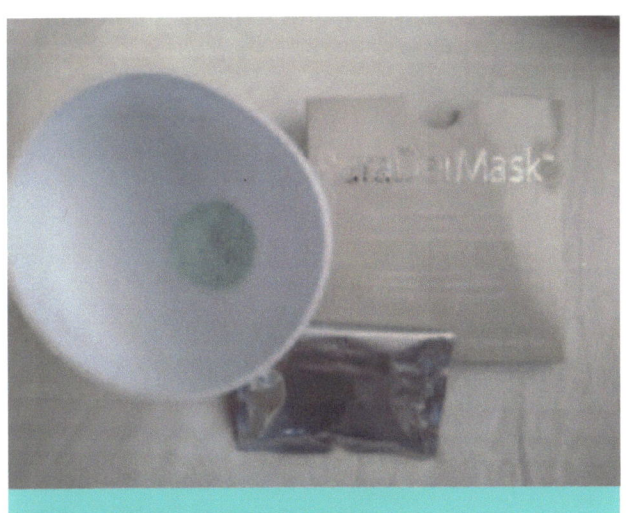

Peel-off patch customizable base compound

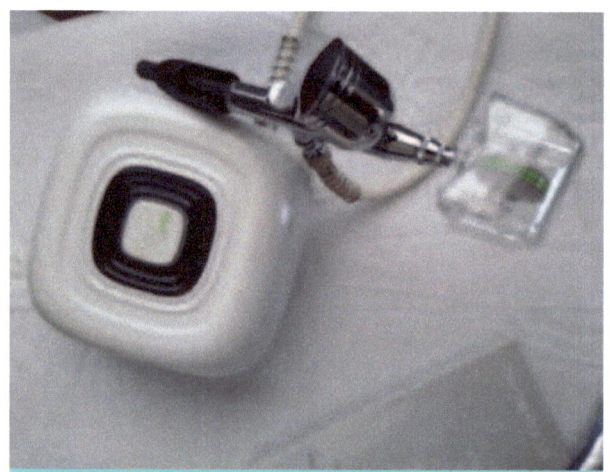

Oxygenated Micro-Mesotherapy device (for negative ionized oxygen and actives infusion)

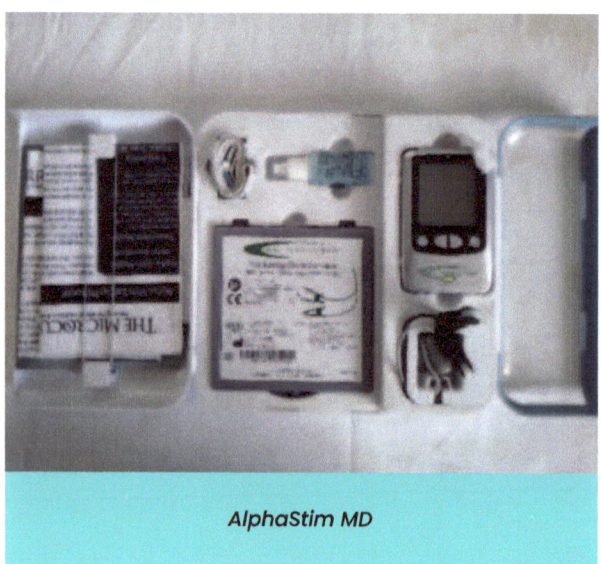

AlphaStim MD

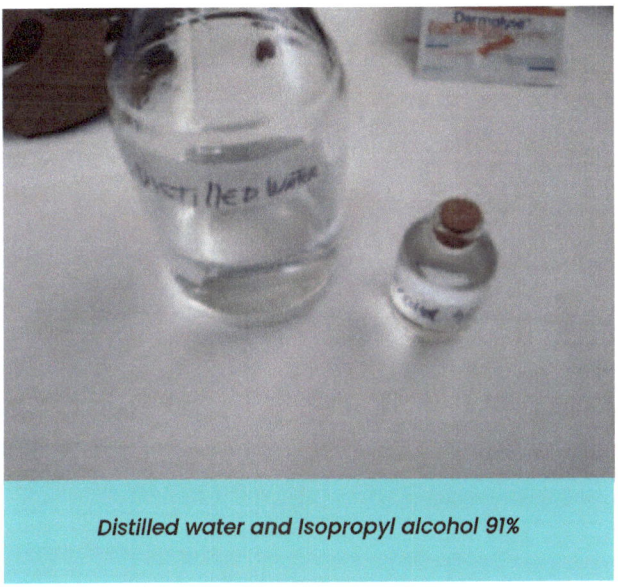

Distilled water and Isopropyl alcohol 91%

Distilled water used for dilution. Isopropyl alcohol 91% used for disinfection.

Note: *Subject will not agree to any procedure involving the injections or needles. No micronutrient testing can be performed as it involves blood collection.*

Duration:

According to Western Herbal Medicine, it will take one month to heal for every year that the ailment has been present.
Typically, if the therapy is effective, an improvement should be noticed in about two weeks. The therapy for this case study will have a duration time of twelve (12) days.

Data Collection and Analysis:
First Data is collected on May 29th.
Next data will be collected on a 6-days basis from the beginning of the therapy – total of 3 treatments.

Breakdown:

Day 1: June 17th – 1st T_x, oral consumption of ad hoc compound, topical application of ad hoc lotion on scar and hands.

Day 2-4: Oral consumption of ad hoc compound, topical application of ad hoc lotion on scar and hands.

Day 5: June 21st – 2nd T_x, oral consumption of ad hoc compound, topical application of ad hoc lotion on scar and hands.

Day 6: June 22nd - Data Collection.

Day 6-8: Oral consumption of ad hoc compound, topical application of ad hoc lotion on scar and hands.

Day 9: June 25th – 3rd T_x, oral consumption of ad hoc compound, topical application of ad hoc lotion on scar and hands.

Day 10-12: Oral consumption of ad hoc compound, topical application of ad hoc lotion on scar and hands.

Day 12: June 28th – AlphaStim T_x.

Day 13: June 29th – Final Data Collection.

On the Final Data Collection, a start/finish comparative analysis will be run to evaluate the performance and results of the proposed therapy: including - but not limited to – 18D Metatron NLS body scan, Quantum Magnetic Resonance (Biochemical Analysis System), before and after pictures of the specific areas addressed.

A personalized therapeutic program is developed in response to the subject's health assessment.

Moderate intensity aerobic exercise is recommended for the stimulation of mitochondrial biogenesis.

The objective is to build oxygen-using capability by conditioning the lungs and heart and by creating oxygen-debt in the muscles. This will stress the mitochondria to send a message to the genes to produce more mitochondria in response (Bland, 2014).

Two compounds are formulated, respectively for oral and topical route. The choice of the form of the remedy is based on several aspects, including the subject's preference, therapy duration and type of condition(s) to treat.

The topical formulation is chosen based on the conditions so far observed, as it allows an easier way to start out. Since there won't be use of needles or other devices for the penetration of the actives, it is essential, to guarantee an effective percutaneous absorption, that the formulation have at least the following characteristics:

- Hydrophilic component
- Lipophilic component
- Molecular weight <500Da

The form of liquid preparation is chosen as a convenient and easy way to administer the remedy internally, for the excellent extracting properties of glycerin and for the unique nutritiousconstituents available in the base used for the compound.

The personalized formulations are designed according to C. Hobbs' theory on the Three (3) Levels of Herbal Activity:

- Deep Immune Activation – herbs main constituents being saponins and complex polysaccharides. Saponins are known to have a strong anti-inflammatory effect (in fact they can be used to synthesize cortisone). These herbs support and strengthen the whole body system with a specific action on the processes having immunity functions – Core Processes of Assimilation/Elimination, Detoxification and Defense.
- Surface Immune Activation – herbs that have pathogen-resistance properties, antimicrobial properties and stimulate the production of

WBCs.
◊ Adaptogens – these herbs act as hormonal modulators, having significant impact on the immunological processes and beneficial effects on the immune response at the level of cellular communication core process.

In conjunction with 3 basic categories of herbs:

◊ Specific/Primary herbs (70-80%) – set the main purpose of the formula, they work directly on the specific ailment/condition.
◊ Supportive & Nourishing herbs (15-20%) – trophorestorative action, these are very high in vitamins and minerals. Soothe and buffer the effects of the other components in the formula.
◊ Activators or Catalyst herbs (10-15%) – have specific effects towards other herbs. These herbs can either stimulate/eliminate or activate the other components in the formula.

The primary focus is put on the mitochondrial functions in relation to external and internal oxidative stress, including the following elements:

♦ **Antioxidants** - Vit.C and Vit. E, to maintain the integrity of cells' structure, antioxidation of lipids in the skin's cellular membrane and counteraction of free radicals.

♦ **Enzymes** - Glutathione Peroxidase, made up of glutamic acid, cysteine and glycine, (a conjugase in the detox process vs. toxins and protection of mitochondria vs. oxygen). SOD (SuperOxideDismutase) and Catalase.

♦ **B-complex** – Vit. B1 (thiamin) regulates carbohydrates metabolism to strengthen the functions of skin, heart and muscles. Vit. B6 (pyridoxine) regulates amino acids metabolism of the nervous system and preserves proper pancreatic functions (conversion of tryptophan to xanthurenic acid).

♦ **Vit. K** – promotes healthy blood coagulation, osmosis, fluid balance regulation and regulate metabolic processes.

♦ **Vit. D3 (cholecalciferol)** – Calcium and phosphorus absorption. Skin protection from UV light.

♦ **Selenium** – carrier of Ca+, concurs to muscle health, especially heart, and immunity. Activates the antioxidant enzymes Glutathione Peroxidase influencing the thyroid secretion as well regulated by the pituitary gland in the anterior lobe.

- **Magnesium** – regulation of the nervous system activity. Preserves the structure of the nucleic acids and protein synthesis. Concurs to muscle contraction. Selenium and Magnesium activate the enzymatic processes in the mitochondria.

Additional support to mitochondrial functions provided by:

- Zinc
- Coenzyme Q10
- Lipoic Acid
- N-acetyl Carnitine
- B2 (riboflavin)
- B3 (niacin)

Objective: Achieve multifunctionality via "more-in-one" approach (Schueller, 2016). pH is kept at 5.35 to maintain protection of the acidic mantle of the skin.

Oral Formulation – liquid extract	Percentage (100mL/g)
Oleum Pini Sibiricae	68%
Glycerin, pure vegetable	5%
Verbena Officinalis, herb	4%
Glycirriza Glabra, root	3%
Harpagophytum Procumbens, root	3%
Nepeta Cataria, herb	3%
Valeriana Officinalis, root	3%
Escholzia Californica, herb	2%
Panax Ginseng, root powder	2%
Aristotelia Chilensis, powder	1%
Centella Asiatica, herb	1%
Hypericum Perforatum, herbal extract	1%
Scutellaria Lateriflora, herbal extract	1%
Sylibum Marianum, herb	1%
Soy Lecithin	1%
Taraxacum Officinale, root	0.6%
Cimicifuga Racemosa, root	0.4%

Aristotelia Chilensis, antioxidant activities on photo ageing of the pores and skin, and inhibition of lipid peroxidation. Delphinidin anthocyanins have antidiabetic properties via inhibition of α-glucosidase, inhibition of pancreatic lipase. Antiviral activities. Prevention of atherosclerosis, promotion of hair growth.

Centella Asiatica, vascular regulatory effect attributed to its saponins. Wound healing properties via Collagen type I synthesis' stimulation.

Cimicifuga Racemosa, emmenagogue and anti-myalgia properties and preventive activity over rheumatoid arthritis. Chemical composition inhibits neutrophil elastase activity and significant increase in bone mineral density.

Escholzia Californica, inhibition of enzymatic degradation and synthesis of adrenaline. It exerts nervine and anxiolytic activity over GI tract, toothaches and rheumatism when combined with ***Valeriana Officinalis***.

Harpagophytum Procumbens, significant analgesic and anti-inflammatory effect thanks to its chemical constituents. Iridoid glycosides – harpagoside, harpagide and procumbide – inhibit lipopolysaccharide-induced iNOS and COX-2 expression via suppression of NF-kB and exert a "bitter" action on the GI tract by increasing gastric acid production and stimulating digestion. Significant action on osteoarthritis prevention via calcium influx regulating mechanisms (Busia, 2016). Ursolic acid, a triterpene, inhibits elastase and MMPs activated by UV rays. Flavonoid kaempferol counteracts collagenase, elastase and hyaluronidase to preserve the ECM. a-sitosterol is immunomodulating and anti-inflammatory.

Hypericum Perforatum, antidepressant activity from the hyposecretion of thyroid hormone, manifesting in mild depression. Sedative effect via the formation of GABA to influence neurotransmitters dopamine an SSRIs. Stimulation of cytochrome P450 -live detox – and P-glycoprotein – detox pathways, in synergy with ***Valeriana Officinalis*** and ***Nepeta Cataria*** they show nervine qualities for stress-induced GI imbalances and anxiolytic actions.

Panax Ginseng, adaptogenic and immunomodulatory properties. Saponins ginsenosides exhibit natural killer cell enhancement and increased immune cell phagocytosis. Improvement on cognitive performance is noted (Busia, 2016).

Sylibum Marianum, chelation properties against MMPs. It contains flavonoids such silybin, silychristin, silydianin. Oral silybin consumption, especially silybin-ß cyclodextrin, protects liver against iron-induced toxicity reduces oxidative and lipid peroxidative damages. Iron binding silybin increase the excretion of heavy metals (Mehrandish, Rahimian & Shahriary, 2019).

Taraxacum Officinale, alterative choleretic and diuretic activities via sesquiterpene lactones, triterpenoids and phytosterols. Rich in Vit. A and C, acid and coumarins. Diuretic activity beneficial for counteracting fluid imbalance and associated oedemas. Hepatic detox functions via action on enzymes CYP1A2 and CYP2E.

Verbena Officinalis, Glycirriza Glabra and ***Scutellaria Lateriflora*** rebuild nervous functions and restore endocrine functions.

Base - Oleum Pini Sibiricae, has a unique chemical composition. Source of B-complex vitamins, especially B1, B2, B3, and fat-soluble vitamin A and D. Tocopherols are present in high levels for an additional antioxidant function. Rich in magnesium and a unique source of minerals like manganese, iron, zinc, calcium, selenium, boron, phosphorus and iodine to support the thyroid gland. High levels of linoleic acid and alpha-linoleic acid to support the cardiovascular system, metabolism and endocrine system regulation. Improves lipids metabolism and lowers cholesterol level while increasing HDL and Apo. In combination with EPA it helps increase and maintain bone mass.

Compound Concentration: 260mg/mL

Note: The natural ingredients in the formulation are have been thoroughly selected based on evidence-based science from thousands of scientific papers accounting for their clinically effective results, safe dosage, side effects and toxicity and complementary adjuncts.
HOWEVER, just because something is natural that doesn't mean that it is safe for everyone. Always check herbs-medications interactions and specific conditions/ailments who may be negatively affected by certain herbal constituents.

Topical Formulation – spray lotion	Percentage (100mL/g)
Distilled Water	30.5%
Aloe Barbadensis, leaf juice	15%
Hamamelis Virginiana, hydroalcoholic extract	10%
Waxes -Natural *Wax Jelly*	10%
Arnica Montana, flower	8%
Antioxidant - *Rubus Chamaemorus*, seed oil	5%
Humectant – *Glycerin*, pure vegetable	4%
Graininess prevention – FSS *Softifan 378*	4%
Emulsifier – *Phytomulse Coconut*	3%
Azadirachta Indica, oil	2.5%
Lavandula Angustifolia, flower	2%
Co-emulsifier – *Soy Lecithin*	2%
Opacifying agent/Thickener – *Stearic Acid*	2%
Preservative – *Optiphen®BSB-W*	1%
Syzygium Aromaticum, oil	1%

Azadirachta Indica, hydrating and antimicrobial properties. Dermatologically used for skin lightening and skin infections.

Arnica Montana, relief of muscle and joint aches and pain via action of its chemical constituents.

Aloe Barbadensis leaf juice, has anti-inflammatory and antiedematous effects. Promotes healing of superficial wounds and skin abrasions by stimulation of the essential matrix components. Reduction of TEWL. Reduction of interleukins productions inducing immunosuppression in keratinocytes. Prevention from UV light damage. Action of glutathione peroxides and SOD on promoting collagen synthesis and counteract free radicals' activity.

Hamamelis Virginiana, astringent, haemostatic and anti-inflammatory actions due to tannins constituents. Hamamelitannins protects skin cells from cellular death from UV rays. Indicated for minor skin injuries, localized inflamed swellings and bruises. Gallic acid has a primary antioxidant free radical scavenging activity. Its flavonoids decrease capillary fragility and permeability. Regulator of sebaceous secretion. Skin barrier protection due to high levels of polyphenolic compounds.

Lavandula Angustifolia, rich in essential oils that have antioxidant and anti-inflammatory activities. Mild nootropic agent.

Rubus Chamaemorus, rich in essential fatty acids, phytosterols and antioxidants. Soothes dry and irritated skin.

Syzygium Aromaticum, antioxidant effects on lipid peroxidation and protein oxidative modification.

Compound Concentration: 435mg/mL
This personalized topical compound is very concentrated and only a small amount is necessary to be applied to the skin and be quickly absorbed completely.

Note: glycosides, lipids, terpenoids, phenols, tannins, alkaloids and flavonoids are biologically available constituents in the plants above mentioned and serve multiple functions to the purpose of the healing process in the FCA™ Model.

"All substances are poisons; there is none which is not a poison. The right dose differentiates a poison or a remedy." - Paracelsus

Regimen

A series of factors concur to determine the adequate dose, amongst these are:

- Concentration mg/mL
- Therapy Duration
- Body Weight/Age
- Sex
- Gender
- Genetic Factors
- Existing Conditions
- Diet and Environment
- Metabolic Disturbances
- Tolerance
- Emotional Factors
- Synergism

Once established a dose for the remedy, the next step is to determine its frequency of use. It is necessary to collect information about rate of absorption, metabolization and elimination:

- Half-life - is the time it takes for the compound to start being eliminated from the body.
- Onset - is the time interval between the administration of the compound and the actual starting of its therapeutic effect. This varies obviously based on the form and route of administration of the remedy.
- Duration of Action – is the length of time during which the therapeutic effect of the compound is manifested.

To establish, up to a certain extent, the most appropriate personalized subject-remedy regimen for the oral liquid compound in this case study, these concurrent factors are considered altogether and a dose, of "best fit" is selected for each active ingredient. The dose is expressed in milligrams (mg).

Respective daily doses of the actives selected from the formula of the oral liquid extract are:

- 170mg
- 320mg
- 120mg
- 4837.5mg
- 1500mg
- 1075mg
- 2000mg
- 1000mg
- 540mg
- 4000mg
- 3000mg
- 2000mg
- 2000mg

For a total amount of 225,625mg.

Divide by 1000 and this amount is converted to grams (g). The proposed result for a daily dose of the liquid extract would be therefore 22.56g, for a concentrated compound of 260mg/mL.

It is obvious to assume that such an amount on a daily basis, for twelve days, would turn out to be anything but safe.
That's when a mild approach to the Law of Minimum Dose can be adopted. Its general notion is that the lower the dose of the remedy, the greater its effectiveness.
What is proposed therefore is to split the total dose over the duration period of the therapy.
22.56g/12days = 1.88g

Since the compound is liquid and therefore expressed in mL and the concentration is in mg/mL, in order to determine the correct dose in mL to be administered the amount in g needs to be converted in mg (1.88x1000 = 1880mg) and then proceed to a simple ratio-proportion calculation.
260mg/1mL = 1880mg/X => 260mgX = 1880mg/mL
Divide both sides by 260mg to obtain the value of the X
260mgX/260mg = X
1880mg/mL /260mg = 7.2mL (approx.)
X=7.2mL
Hence the daily dose would be 7.2mL, which can be conveniently consumed as 3.6mL twice a day (bid).

Protocol

Tx₁ – June 17ᵗʰ

Mechano-chemical peeling gel 0.5mL, 3 minute action on site and removal using sponge an distilled water.

Mesocomplex Actives formulation 0.5mL, dilution ratio 1:1 w/ distilled water; introduce in the tank of Oxygenated Micro-Mesotherapy device for negative ionized oxygen and actives infusion.

Procedure on high pressure and micropin head 198 pins, size 0.5mm.

Duration of the procedure 5 minutes.

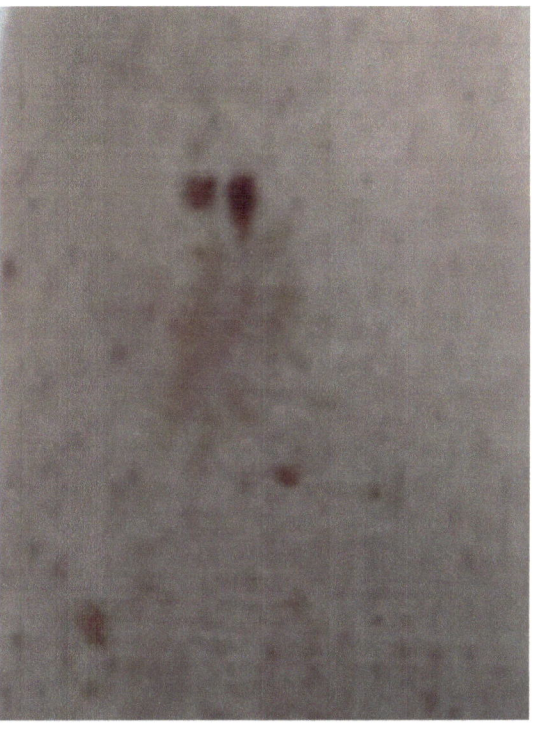

Application of personalized topical lotion 1.15mL on scarred area and 0.6mL per hand - bid. via occlusive application of peel-off base compound to increase absorption rate. Duration 15 minutes.

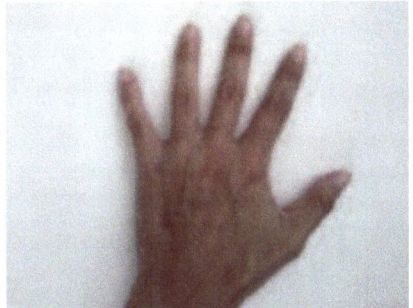 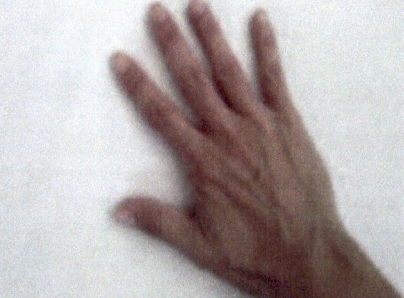

Application of multiactive viscoelastic cream-gel, filmogenic effect. Oral consumption 3.6mL personalized liquid extract - bid ac.

Tx_2 – June 21st

Mechano-chemical peeling gel 0.5mL, 3 minute action on site and removal using sponge an distilled water.

Mesocomplex Actives formulation 0.5mL, dilution ratio 1:1 w/ distilled water; introduce in the tank of Oxygenated Micro-Mesotherapy device for negative ionized oxygen and actives infusion.

Procedure on high pressure and micropin head 198 pins, size 0.5mm. Duration of the procedure 5 minutes.

Application of personalized topical lotion 1.15mL on scarred area and 0.6mL per hand bid. via occlusive application of peel-off base compound to increase absorption rate. Duration 15 minutes.

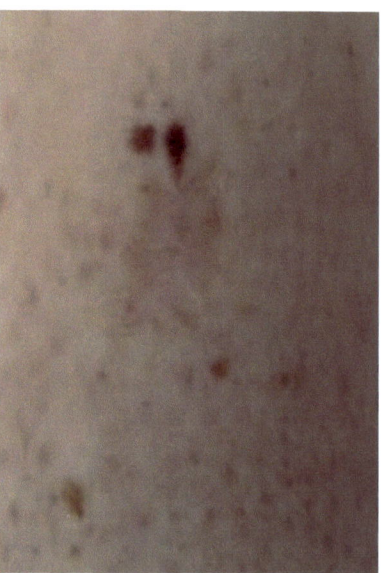

Application of Woven-leaf Herbal patch (Camelia Sinensis Leaf, Mentha Piperita Leaf), 15 minutes.

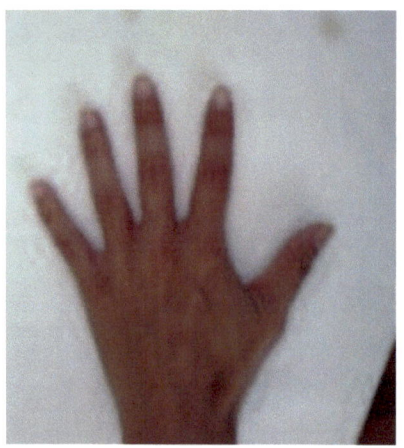
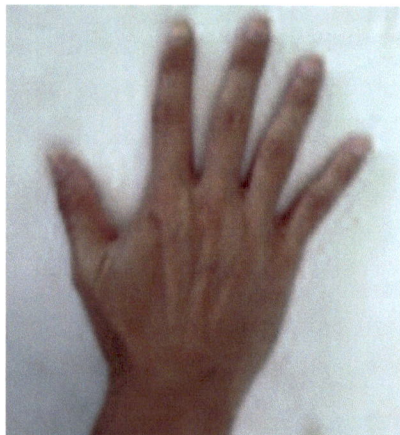

Application of multiactive viscoelastic cream-gel, filmogenic effect. Oral consumption 3.6mL personalized liquid extract bid ac.

Tx₃ – June 25ᵗʰ

Mechano-chemical peeling gel 0.5mL, 3 minute action on site and removal using sponge an distilled water.

Mesocomplex Actives formulation 0.5mL, dilution ratio 1:1 w/ distilled water; introduce in the tank of Oxygenated MicroMesotherapy device for negative ionized oxygen and actives infusion.

Procedure on high pressure and micropin head 198 pins, size 0.5mm.

Duration of the procedure 5 minutes.

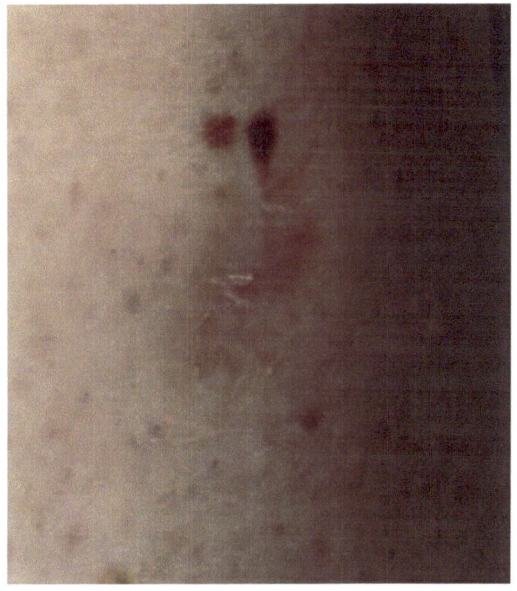

Application of personalized topical lotion 1.15mL on scarred area and 0.6mL per hand bid. via occlusive application of peel-off base compound to increase absorption rate. Duration 15 minutes.

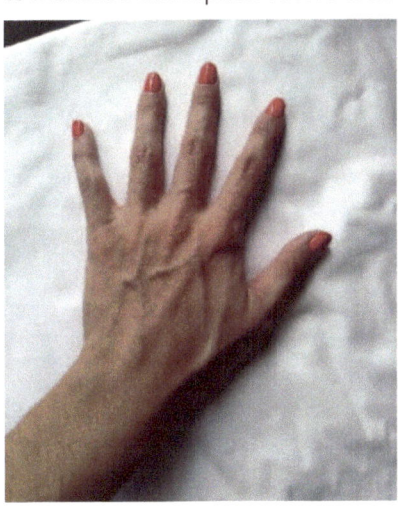
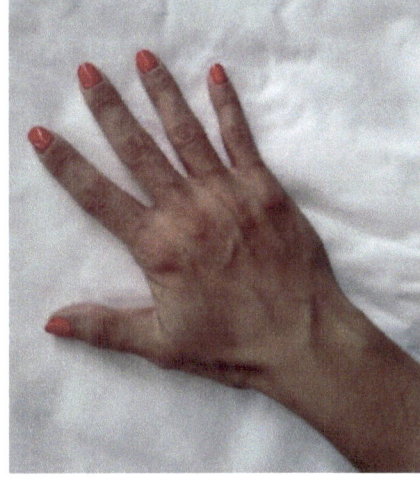

Application of Woven-leaf Herbal patch (Camelia Sinensis Leaf, Mentha Piperita Leaf), 15 minutes.

Application of multiactive viscoelastic cream-gel, filmogenic effect.

Oral consumption 3.6mL personalized liquid extract bid ac.

AlphaStim MD, duration 20 minutes, power 4.5

CHAPTER FIVE
Comparative Findings

Note: *The test results are intended as reference only and not as a diagnostic conclusion.*

Magnetic Resonance Quantum Analyzer WF-QA46

Test Report 06/03/2020 vs 06/22/2020

https://qrgo.page.link/yD8QG

https://qrgo.page.link/KpEKz

- Pancreatic function – slight increase of insulin level.

- Bones degeneration: adhesion degree of shoulder muscle from u.012 to u.0.24 (optimal is < u 0.2) slight improvement of aging of ligaments from 22% to 21%.

- Trace minerals; deficiency of potassium levels.

- Coenzyme; deficiency of Glutathione levels.

- Toxin; mildly high levels of tobacco/nicotine.

- Heavy Metals; mildly high antimony levels.

- Pulse heart and brain; Stroke Volume (SV) from mildly deficient function to optimal values, Pulse wave coefficient K from normal values to mild deficiency.

18D Metatron NLS

Test Report 05/29/2020 vs 06/22/2020

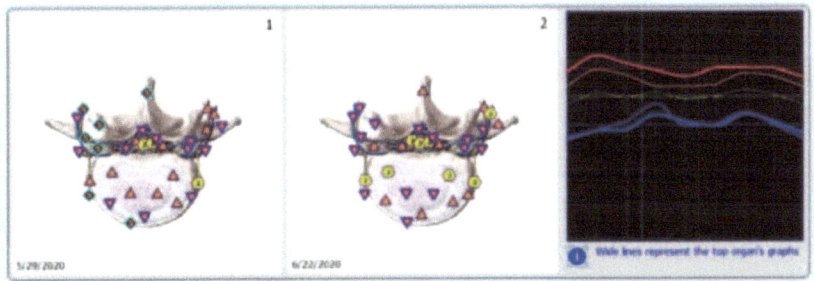

Strengthening compensatory reactions 34%
5/29/2020 First Lumbar vertebra

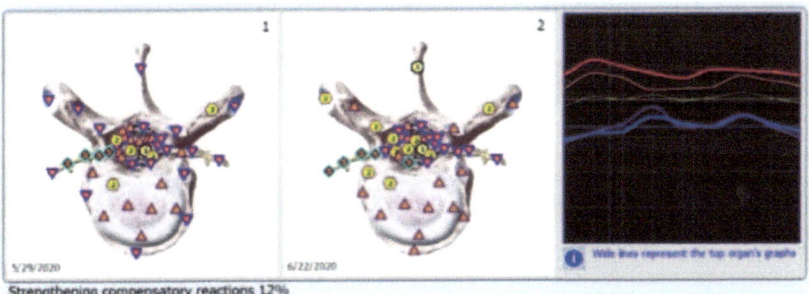

Strengthening compensatory reactions 12%
5/29/2020 First thoracic vertebra

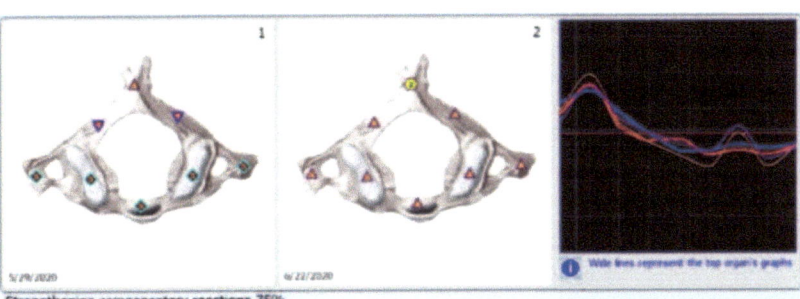

Strengthening compensatory reactions 75%
5/29/2020 Second neck-bone

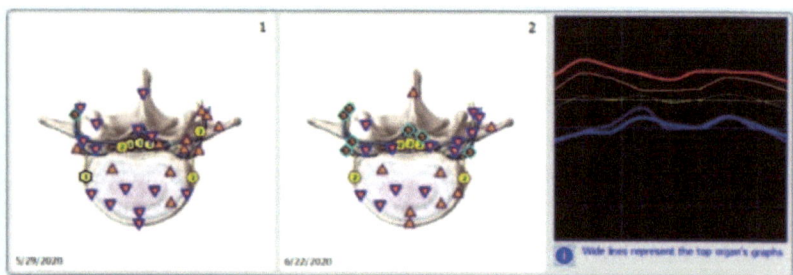
Weakening compensatory reactions 31%
5/29/2020 Second lumbar vertebra

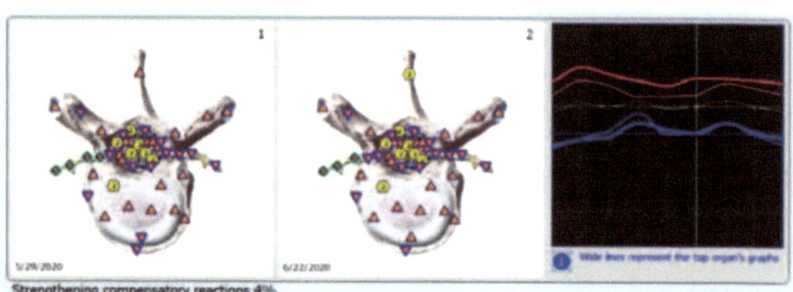
Strengthening compensatory reactions 4%
5/29/2020 Second thoracic vertebra

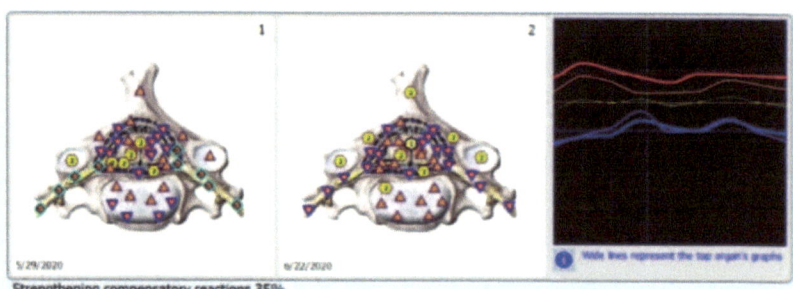
Strengthening compensatory reactions 35%
5/29/2020 Third neck-bone

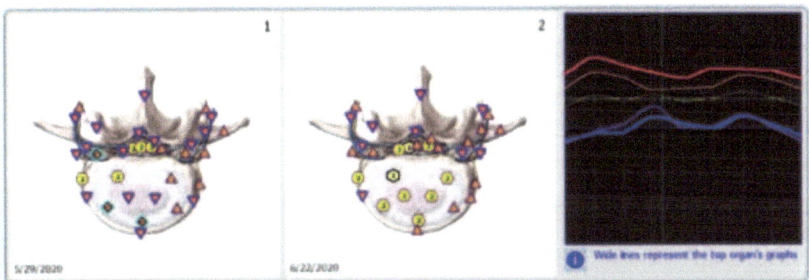

Strengthening compensatory reactions 39%
5/29/2020 Third lumbar vertebra

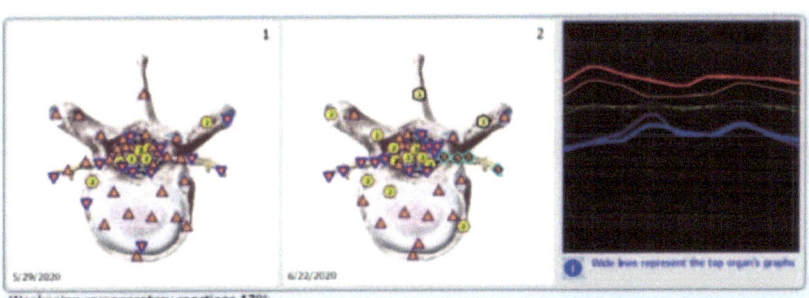

Weakening compensatory reactions 13%
5/29/2020 Third thoracic vertebra

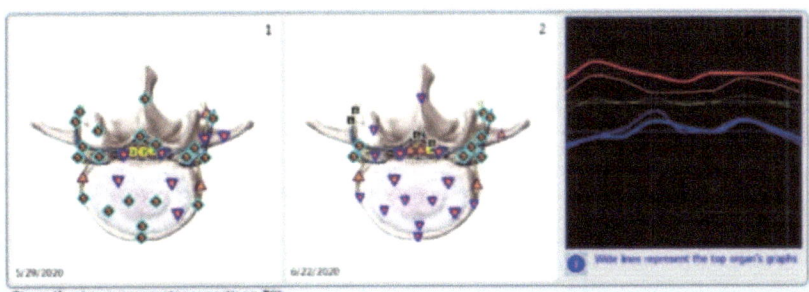

Strengthening compensatory reactions 3%
Increasing of nidus of defeat by 100%
5/29/2020 Fourth lumbar vertebra

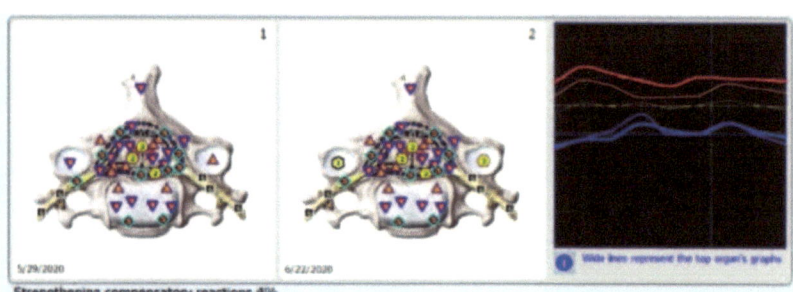

Strengthening compensatory reactions 4%
Nidus of defeat without changes
5/29/2020 Fourth neck-bone

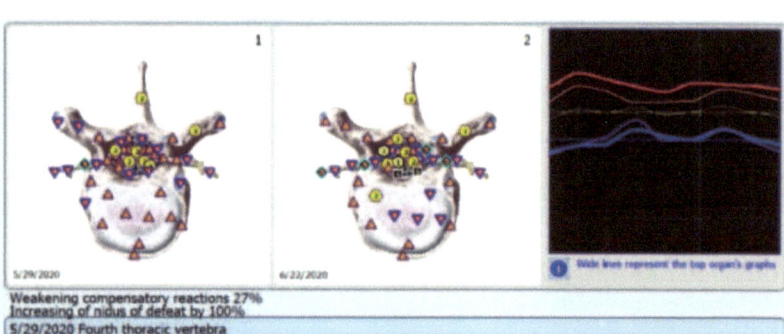

Weakening compensatory reactions 27%
Increasing of nidus of defeat by 100%
5/29/2020 Fourth thoracic vertebra

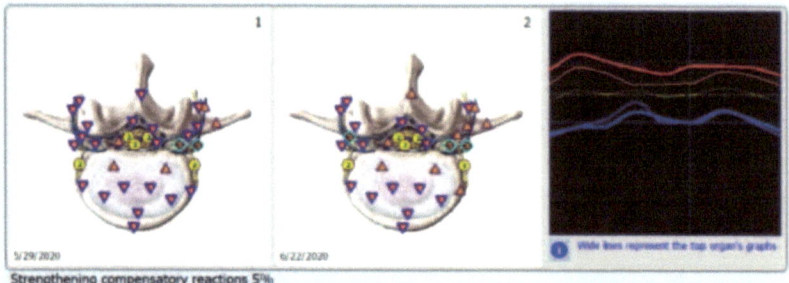

Strengthening compensatory reactions 5%
5/29/2020 Fifth lumbar vertebra

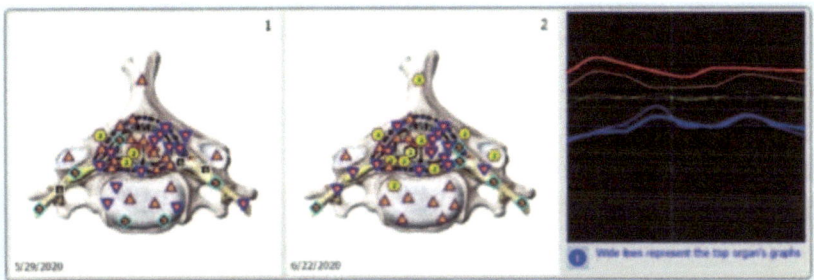

Strengthening compensatory reactions 28%
Decreasing of nidus of defeat by 100%
5/29/2020 Fifth neck-bone

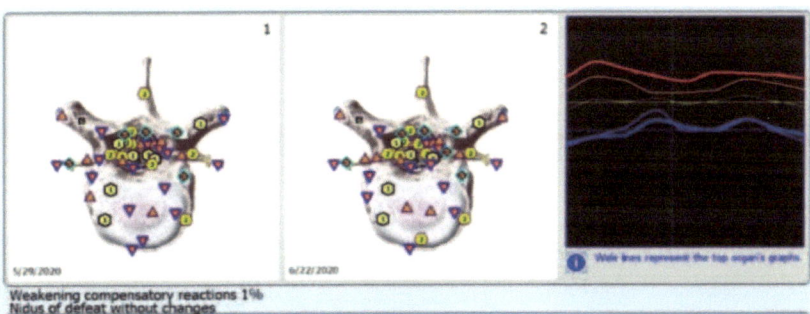

Weakening compensatory reactions 1%
Nidus of defeat without changes
5/29/2020 Fifth thoracic vertebra

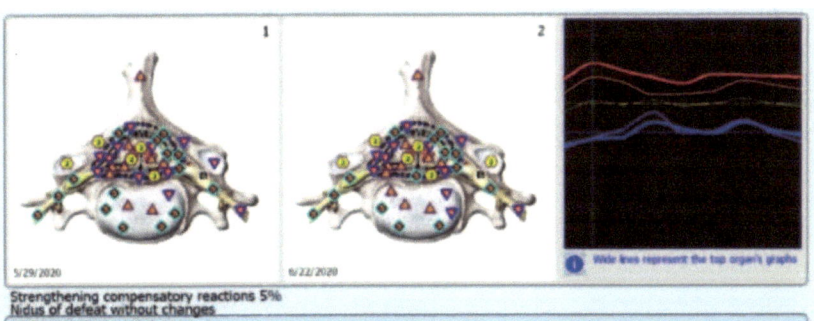

Strengthening compensatory reactions 5%
Nidus of defeat without changes
5/29/2020 Sixth neck-bone

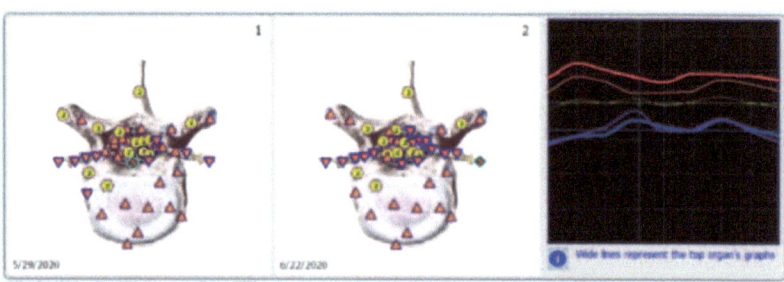

Weakening compensatory reactions 18%
5/29/2020 Sixth thoracic vertebra

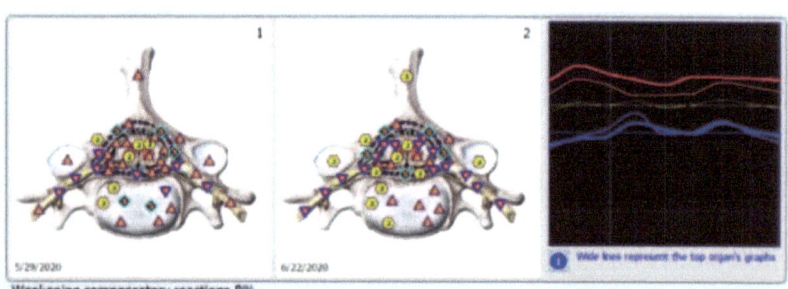

Weakening compensatory reactions 8%
5/29/2020 Seventh neck-bone

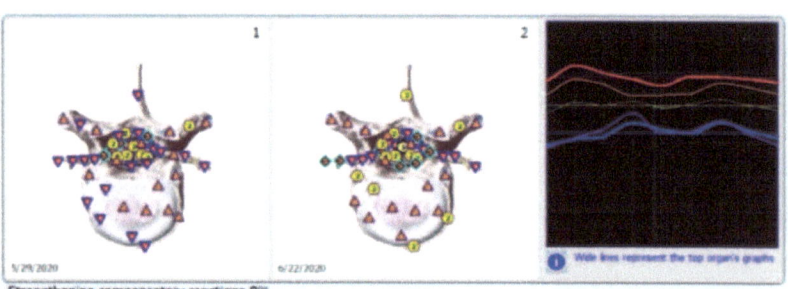

Strengthening compensatory reactions 8%
5/29/2020 Seventh thoracic vertebra

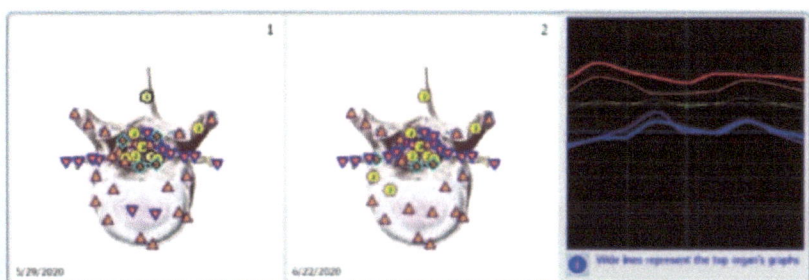

Strengthening compensatory reactions 1%
5/29/2020 Ninth thoracic vertebra

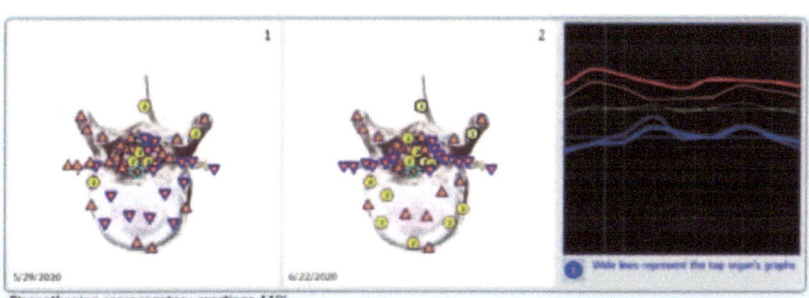

Strengthening compensatory reactions 11%
5/29/2020 Tenth thoracic vertebra

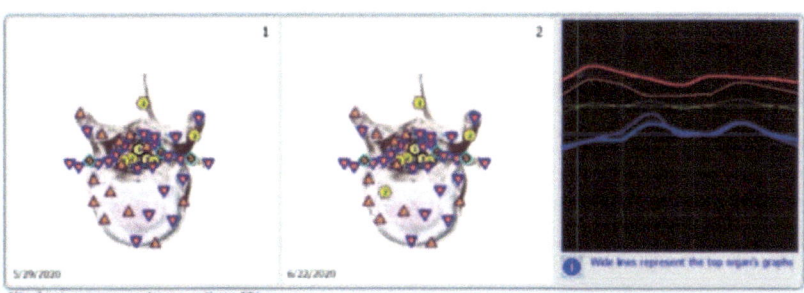

Weakening compensatory reactions 1%
5/29/2020 Eleventh thoracic vertebra

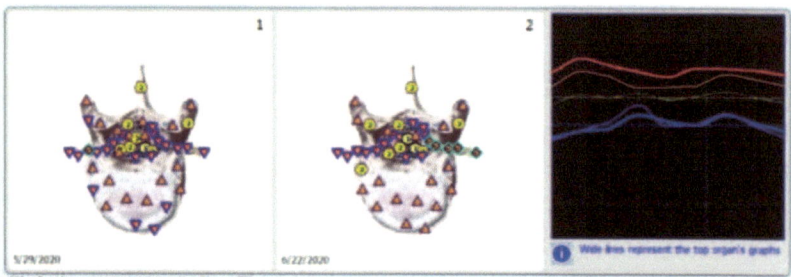

Weakening compensatory reactions 4%
5/29/2020 Twelfth thoracic vertebra

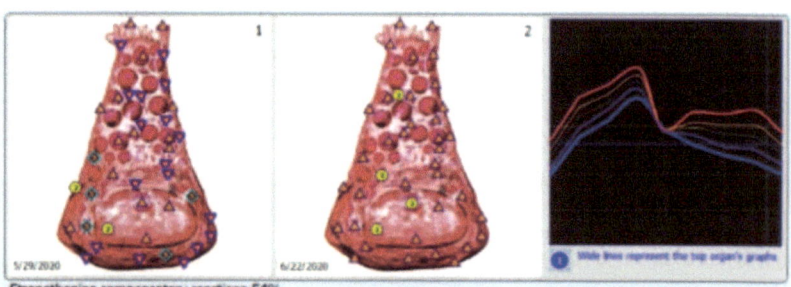

Strengthening compensatory reactions 54%
5/29/2020 Acinic insular cells of pancreas

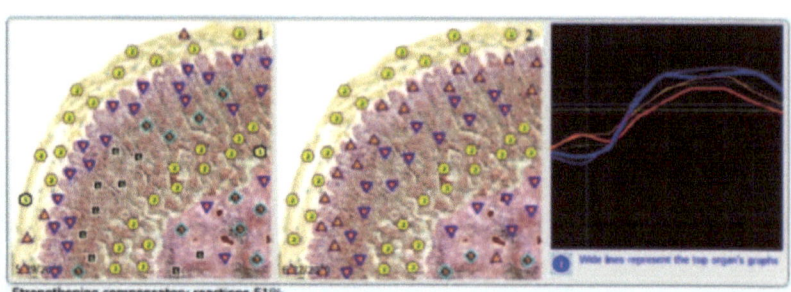

Strengthening compensatory reactions 51%
Decreasing of nidus of defeat by 100%
5/29/2020 Adrenal

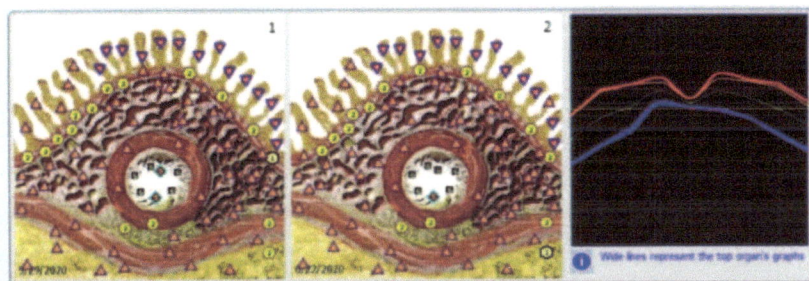

Weakening compensatory reactions 2%
Increasing of nidus of defeat by 17%
5/29/2020 Ampulla of vater duct

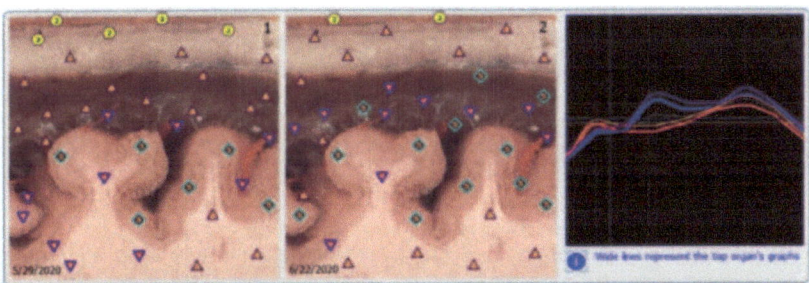

Weakening compensatory reactions 25%
5/29/2020 Arachnoid membrane

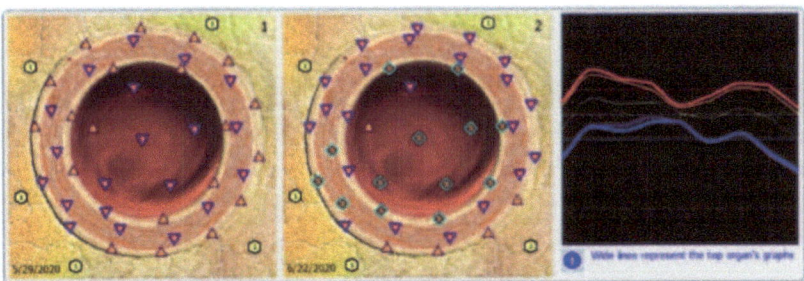

Weakening compensatory reactions 42%
5/29/2020 Arteria

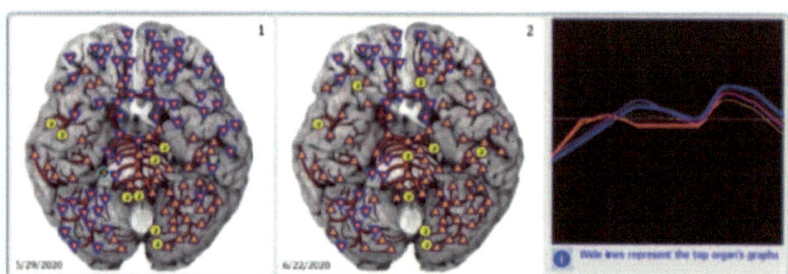

Strengthening compensatory reactions 22%
5/29/2020 Arteries of brain:view from below

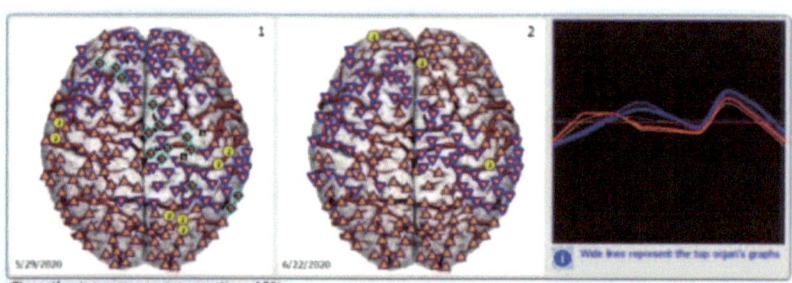

Strengthening compensatory reactions 16%
Decreasing of nidus of defeat by 100%
5/29/2020 Arteries of cerebrum:view from above

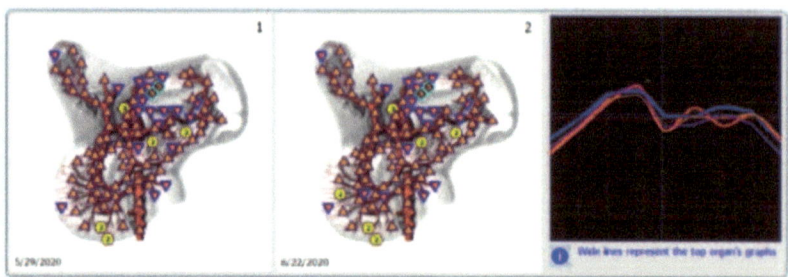

Strengthening compensatory reactions 1%
5/29/2020 Arteries of duodenum and pancreas

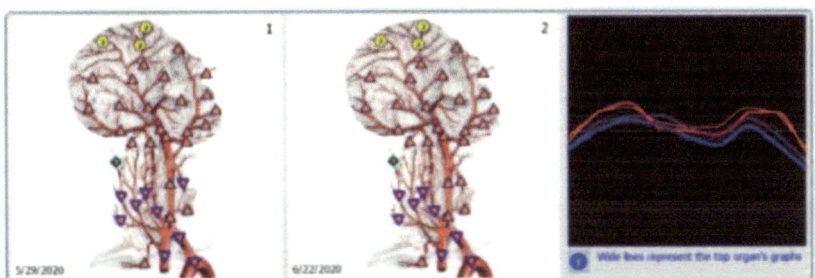

Strengthening compensatory reactions 3%
5/29/2020 Arteries of head and neck:right view

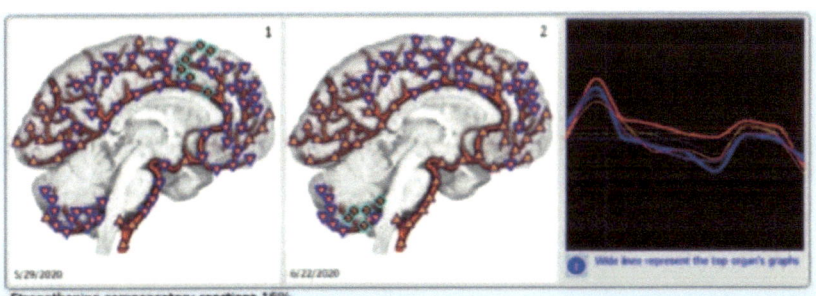

Strengthening compensatory reactions 16%
5/29/2020 Arteries of the medial surface of cerebrum:left view

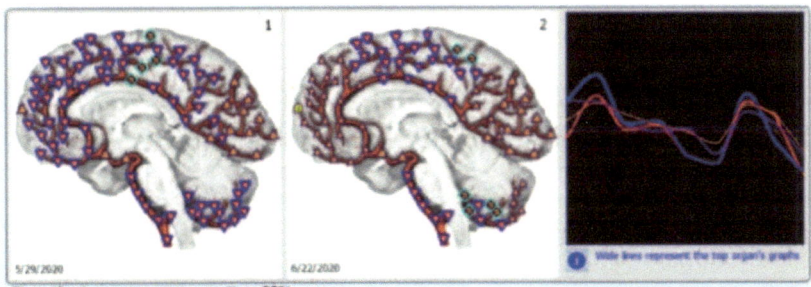

Strengthening compensatory reactions 23%
5/29/2020 Arteries of the medial surface of cerebrum:right view

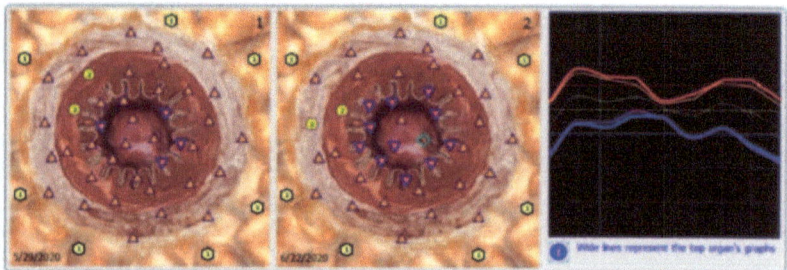

Weakening compensatory reactions 23%
5/29/2020 Arteriola

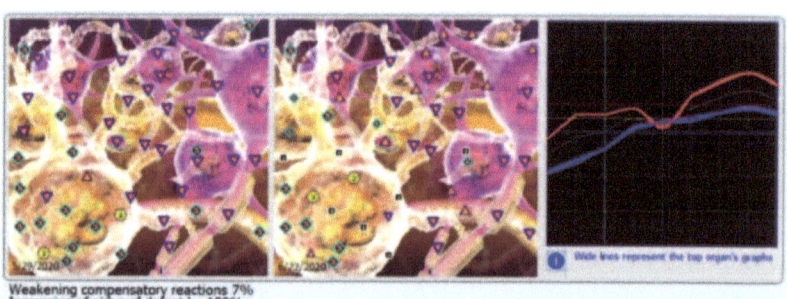

Weakening compensatory reactions 7%
Increasing of nidus of defeat by 100%
5/29/2020 Astrocytes

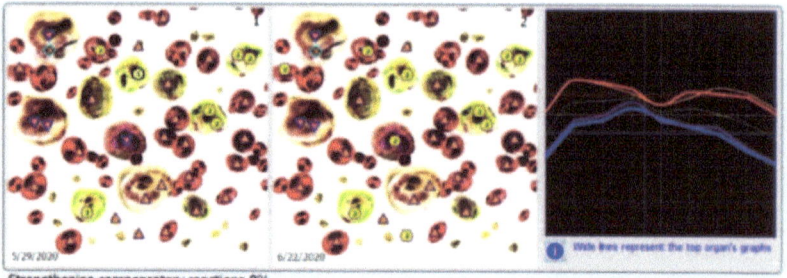

Strengthening compensatory reactions 8%
5/29/2020 Blood cells

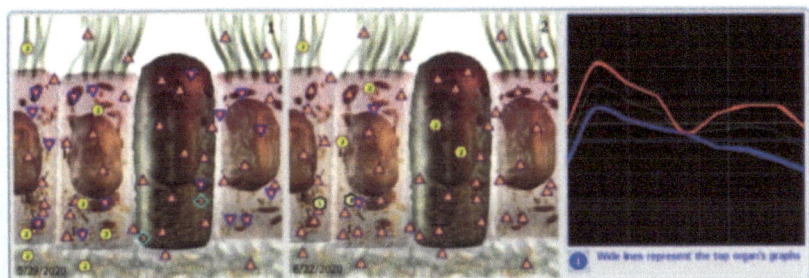
Strengthening compensatory reactions 32%
5/29/2020 Bronchiolar epithelium

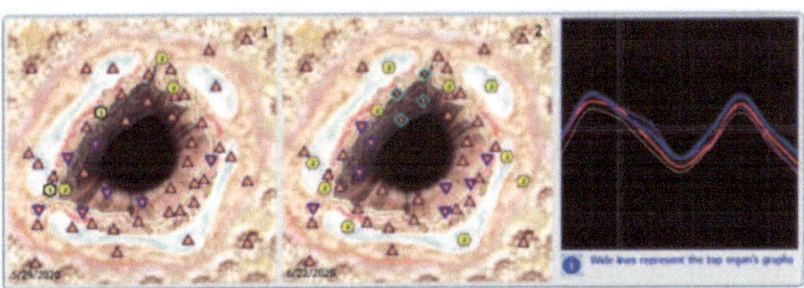
Weakening compensatory reactions 18%
5/29/2020 Bronchus cut

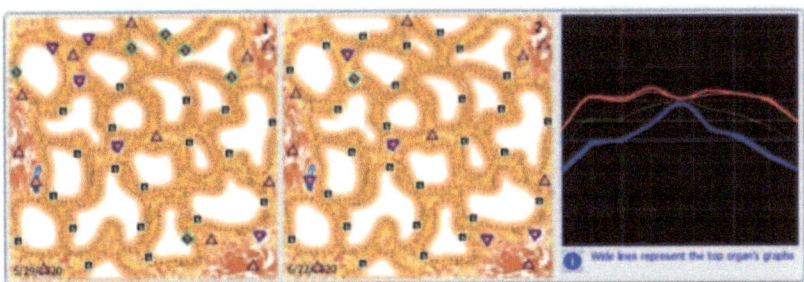
Weakening compensatory reactions 16%
Increasing of nidus of defeat by 30%
5/29/2020 Bulbourethral glands

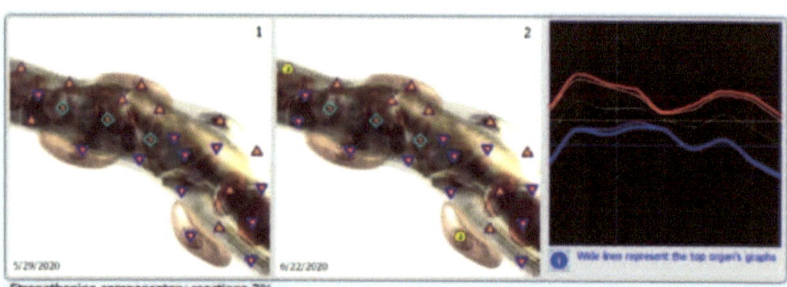
5/29/2020 Capillar

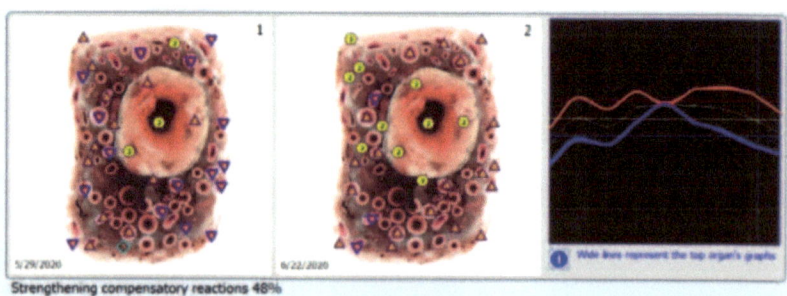
5/29/2020 Cells of fascicular region

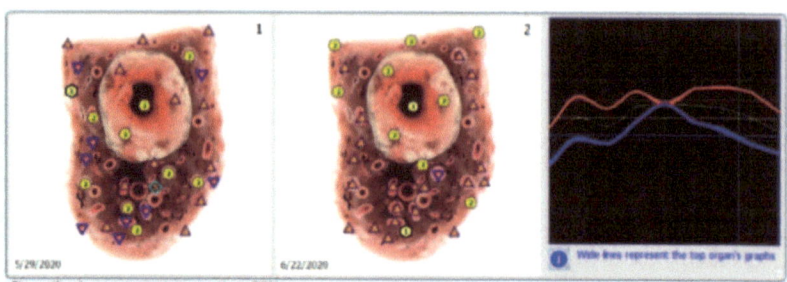
5/29/2020 Cells of glomerular region

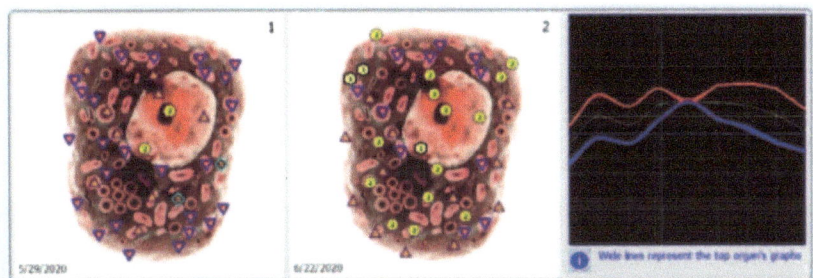

Strengthening compensatory reactions 48%
5/29/2020 Cells of reticular region

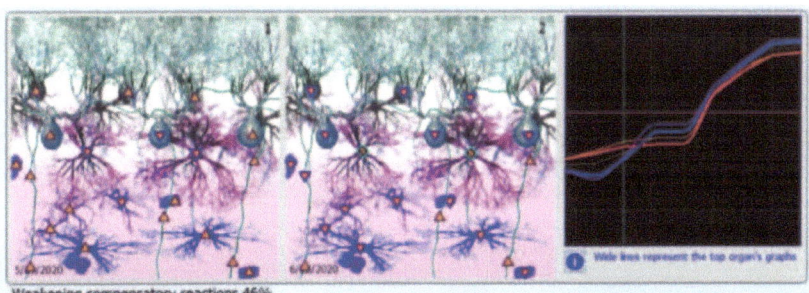

Weakening compensatory reactions 46%
5/29/2020 Cerebellum tissue

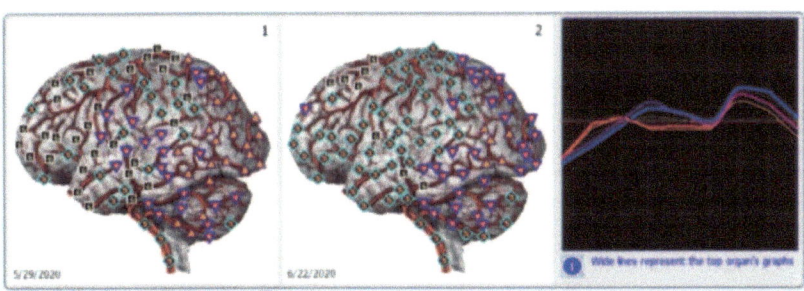

Strengthening compensatory reactions 5%
Decreasing of nidus of defeat by 71%
5/29/2020 Cerebral arteries: lateral view of left hemisphere

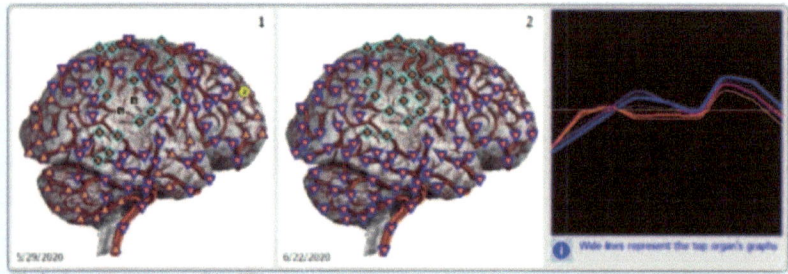

Weakening compensatory reactions 16%
Decreasing of nidus of defeat by 100%
5/29/2020 Cerebral arteries:lateral view of right hemisphere

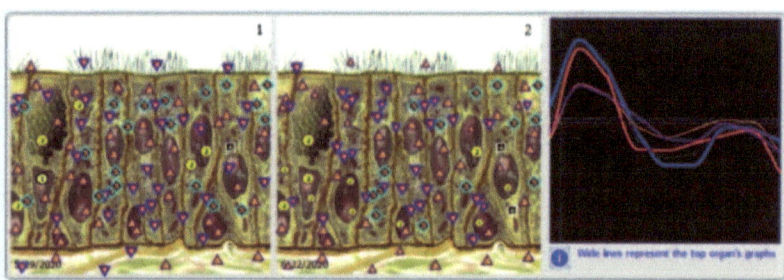

Strengthening compensatory reactions 10%
Increasing of nidus of defeat by 50%
5/29/2020 Ciliated epithelial cell

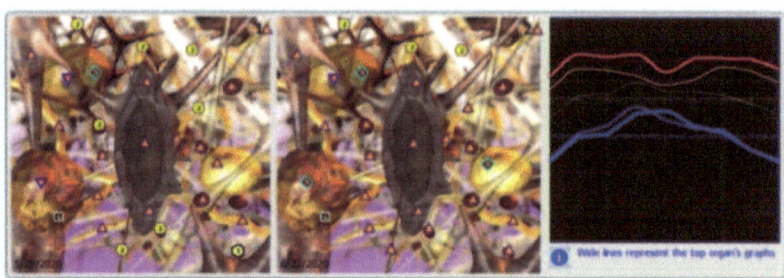

Weakening compensatory reactions 22%
Nidus of defeat without changes
5/29/2020 Connective tissue

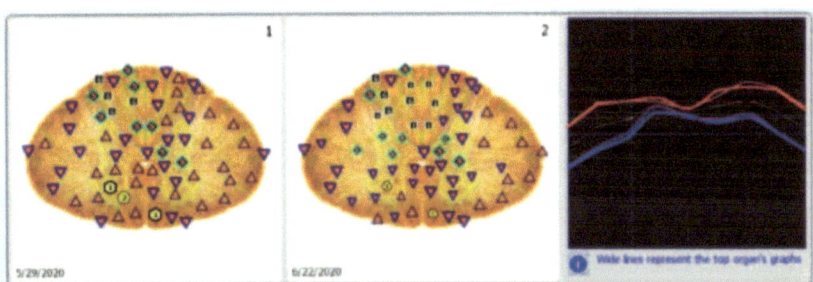

Weakening compensatory reactions 28%
Increasing of nidus of defeat by 60%
5/29/2020 Cross section of spinal cord

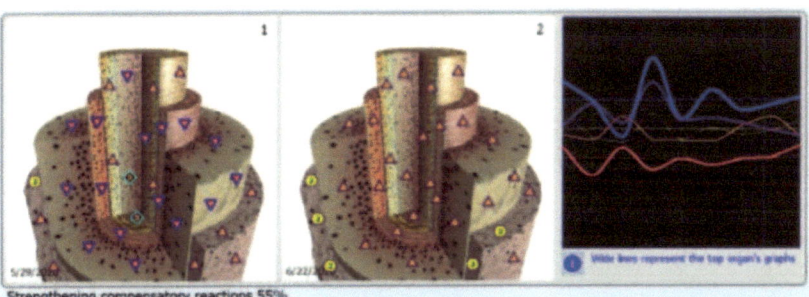

Strengthening compensatory reactions 55%
5/29/2020 Cuticle of hair

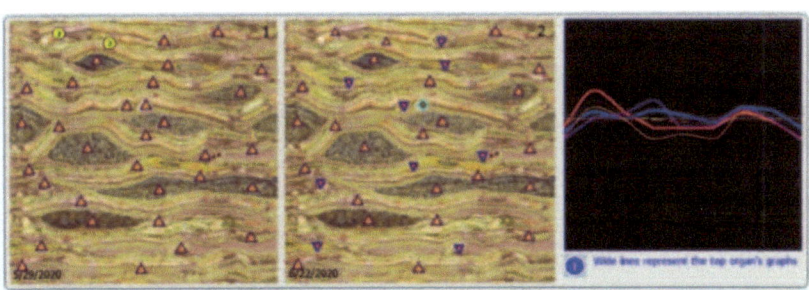

Weakening compensatory reactions 35%
5/29/2020 Dense non-formed connective tissue

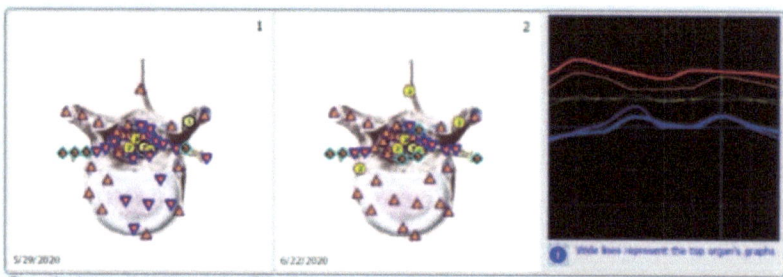

Strengthening compensatory reactions 8%
5/29/2020 Eight thoracic vertebra

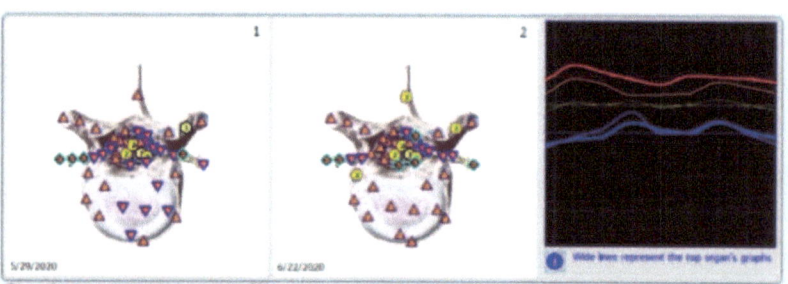

Strengthening compensatory reactions 8%
5/29/2020 Eight thoracic vertebra

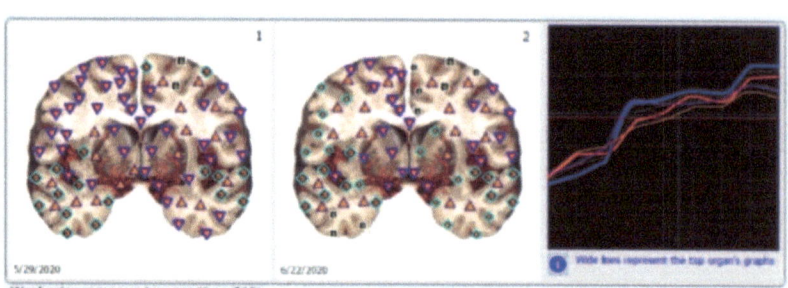

Weakening compensatory reactions 21%
Increasing of nidus of defeat by 78%
5/29/2020 Encephalon arteries,crown section

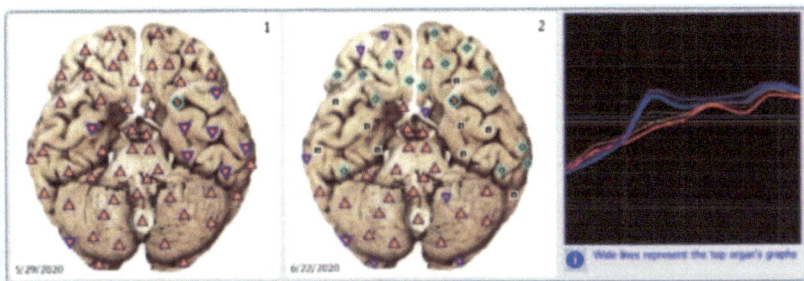

Weakening compensatory reactions 63%
Increasing of nidus of defeat by 100%
5/29/2020 Encephalon, cranial nerves: bottom view

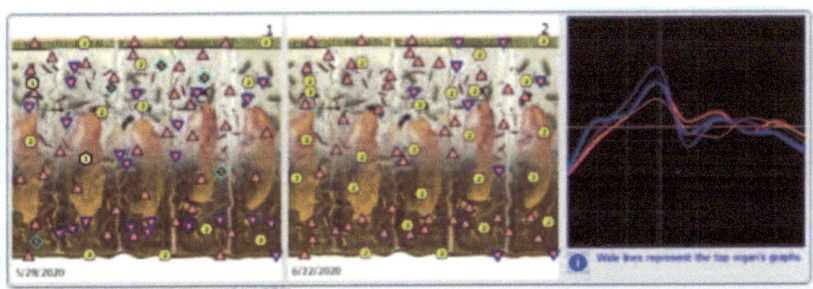

Strengthening compensatory reactions 38%
5/29/2020 Epithelial cell of intestine

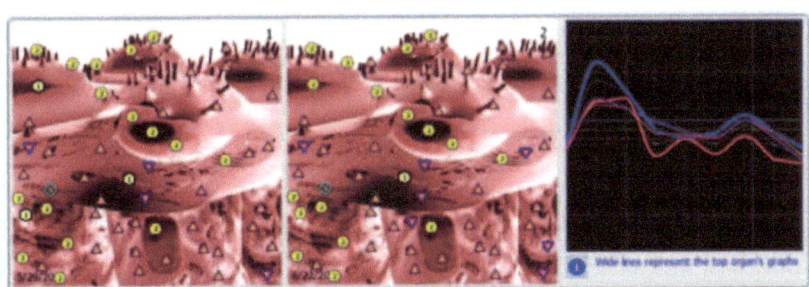

Weakening compensatory reactions 9%
5/29/2020 Endothelial cells

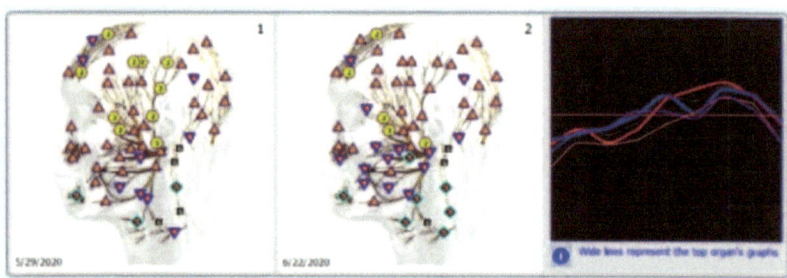
Weakening compensatory reactions 15%
Decreasing of nidus of defeat by 25%
5/29/2020 Facial nerve:left view

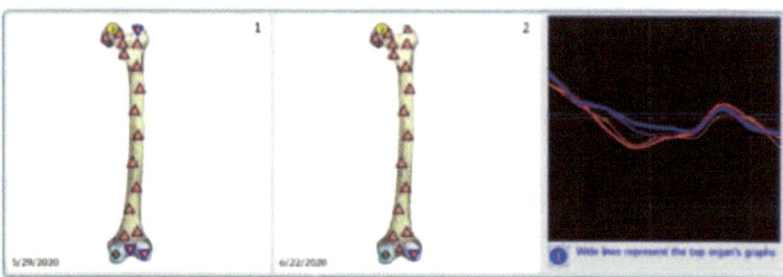
Strengthening compensatory reactions 11%
5/29/2020 Femur:right

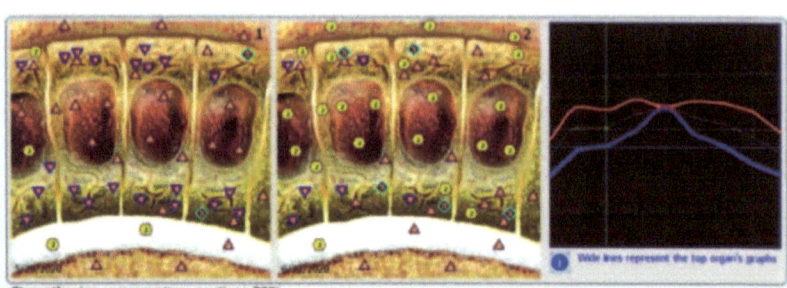
Strengthening compensatory reactions 26%
5/29/2020 Follicular ovary cells

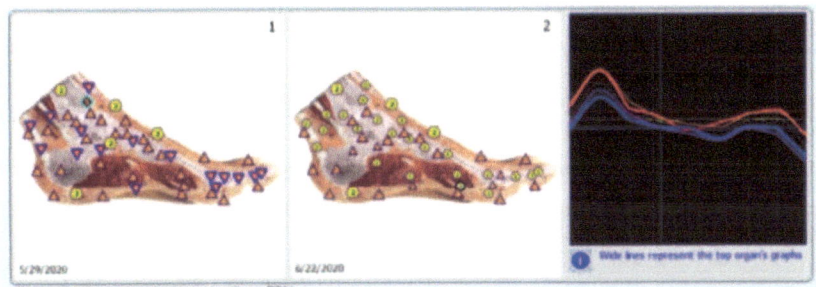

Strengthening compensatory reactions 58%
5/29/2020 Foot cut:left view

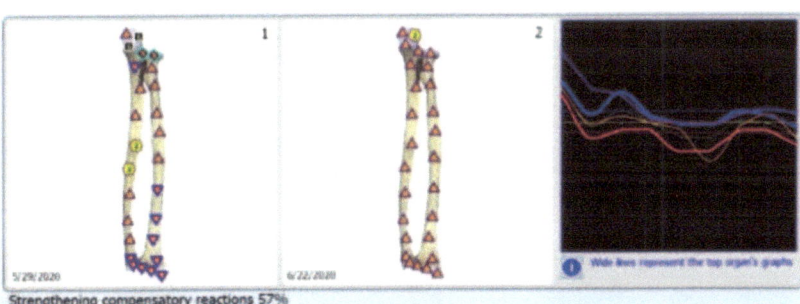

Strengthening compensatory reactions 57%
Decreasing of nidus of defeat by 100%
5/29/2020 Forearm bones:left view

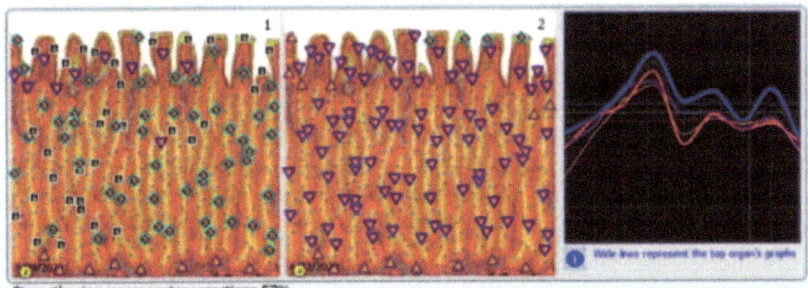

Strengthening compensatory reactions 57%
Decreasing of nidus of defeat by 100%
5/29/2020 Gastric glands

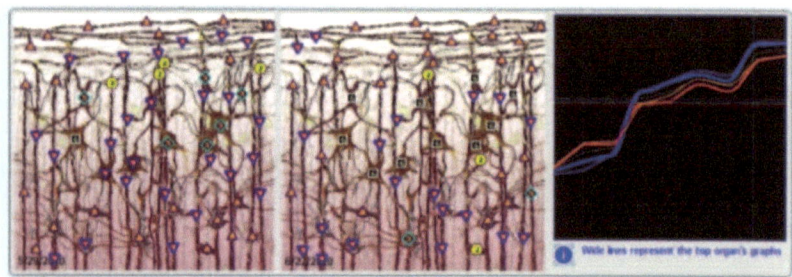
Weakening compensatory reactions 25%
Increasing of nidus of defeat by 90%
5/29/2020 Gray matter of cerebrum

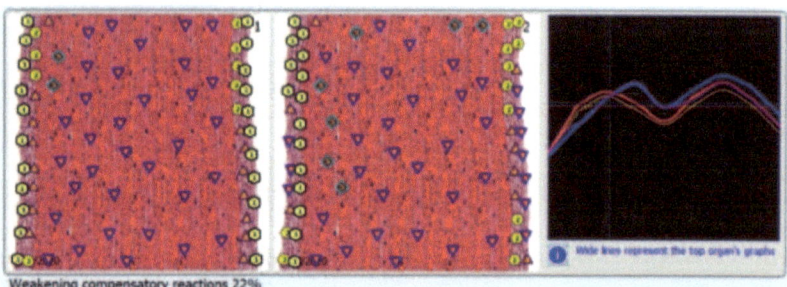
Weakening compensatory reactions 22%
5/29/2020 Interventricular septum

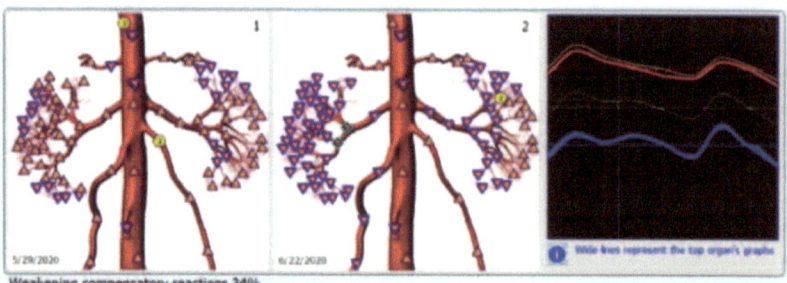
Weakening compensatory reactions 34%
5/29/2020 Kidney vessels

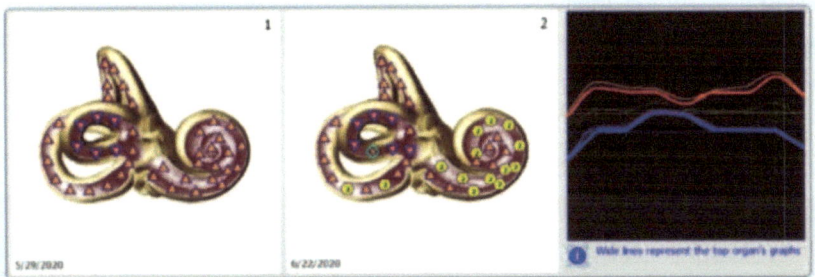
Strengthening compensatory reactions 12%
5/29/2020 Labyrinth:right view

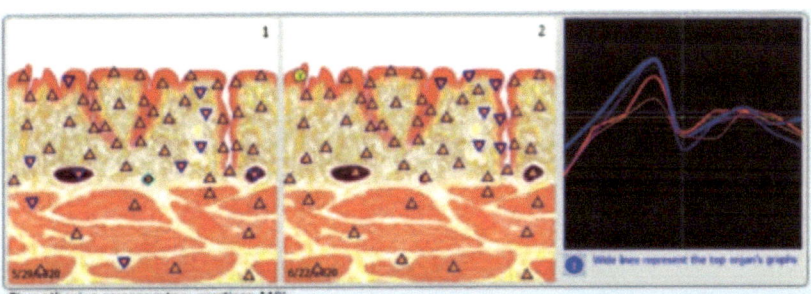
Strengthening compensatory reactions 11%
5/29/2020 Lingual papilla

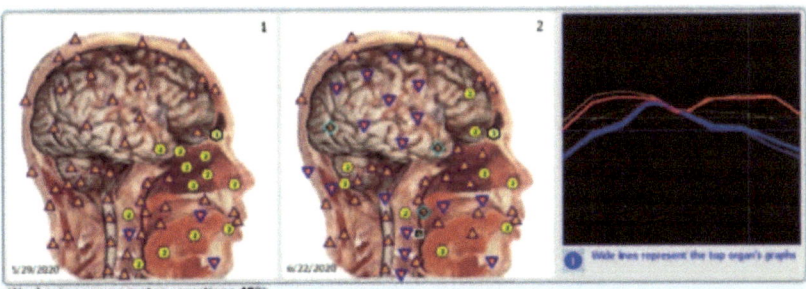
Weakening compensatory reactions 40%
Increasing of nidus of defeat by 100%
5/29/2020 Longitudinal cross-section of head:right view

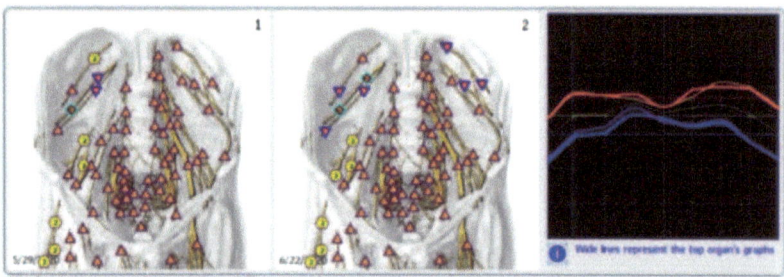

Weakening compensatory reactions 11%
5/29/2020 Lumbosacral plexus

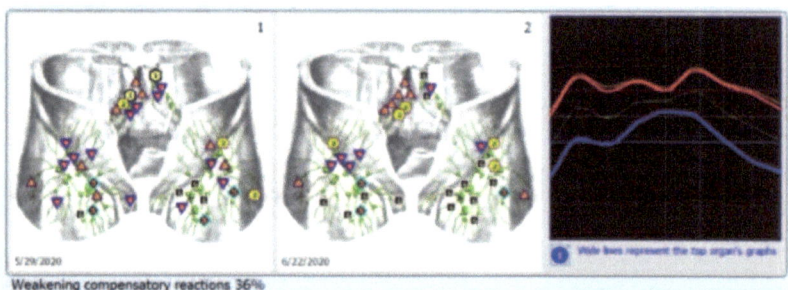

Weakening compensatory reactions 36%
Increasing of nidus of defeat by 69%
5/29/2020 Lymphatic nodes in inguinal part

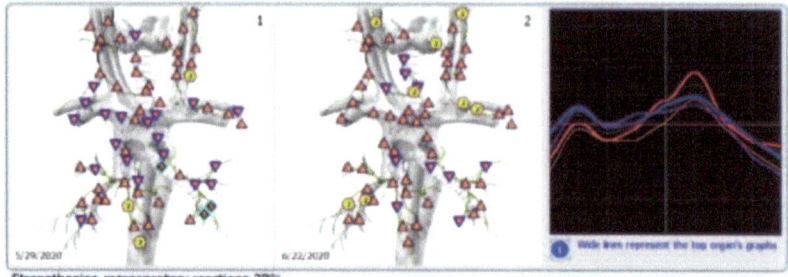

Strengthening compensatory reactions 28%
5/29/2020 Lymphatic vessels of mediastinum

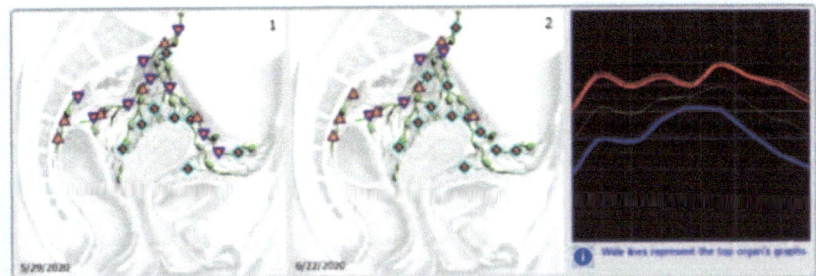
Weakening compensatory reactions 11%
5/29/2020 Lymphatic vessels of pelvis: left view

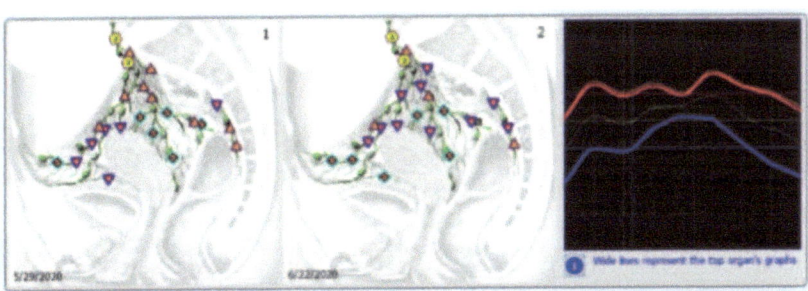
Weakening compensatory reactions 19%
Increasing of nidus of defeat by 100%
5/29/2020 Lymphatic vessels of pelvis: right view

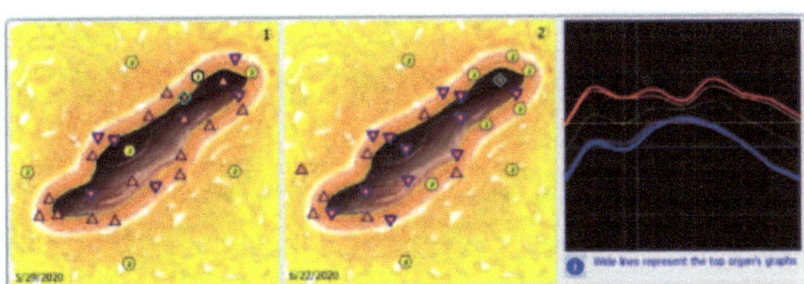
Weakening compensatory reactions 17%
5/29/2020 Lymphatic vessel

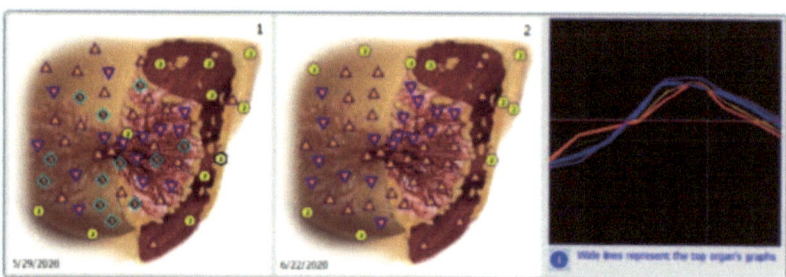
Strengthening compensatory reactions 34%
5/29/2020 Mammary gland duct:left view

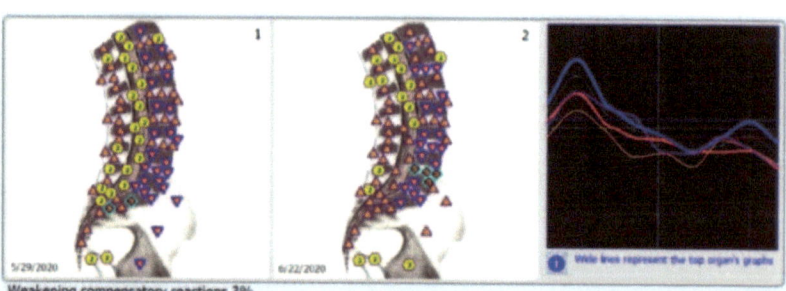
Weakening compensatory reactions 3%
5/29/2020 Median sagittal section of inferior sector of vertebral column:right view

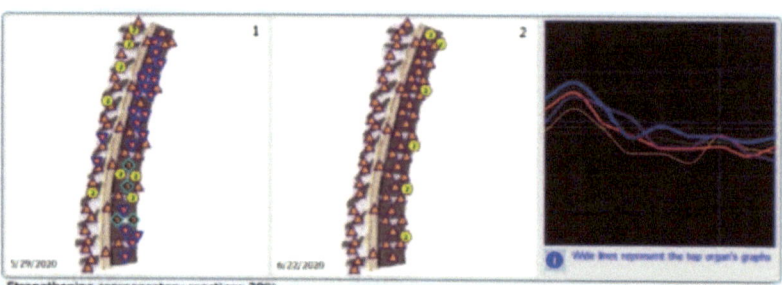
Strengthening compensatory reactions 39%
5/29/2020 Median sagittal section of thoracic vertebrae:left view

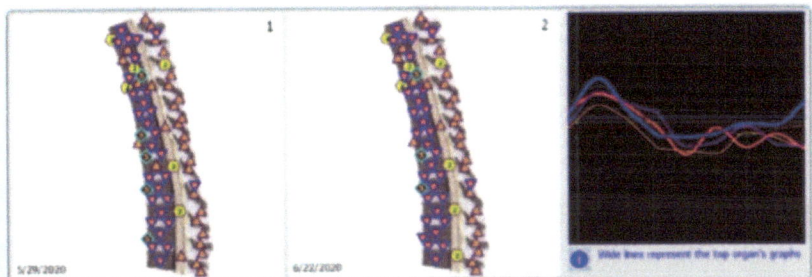

Strengthening compensatory reactions 3%

5/29/2020 Median sagittal section of thoracic vertabrae:right view

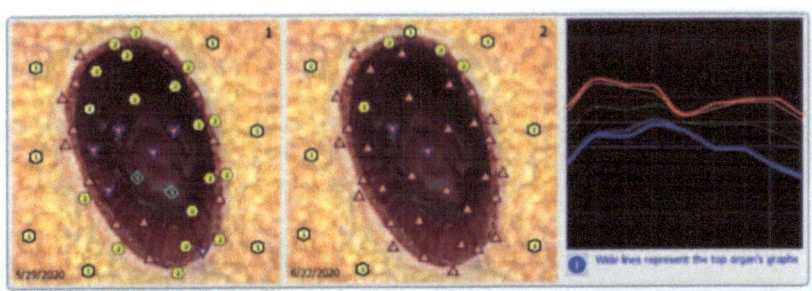

Strengthening compensatory reactions 9%

5/29/2020 Medium calibre vein

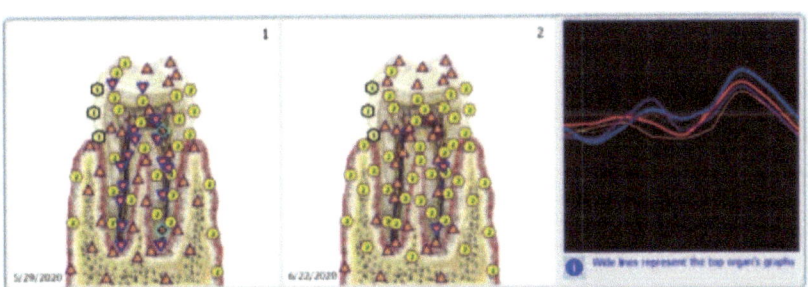

Strengthening compensatory reactions 44%

5/29/2020 Molar tooth

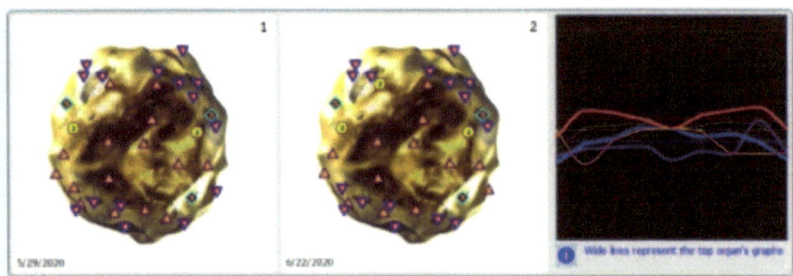
Weakening compensatory reactions 1%
5/29/2020 Monocyte

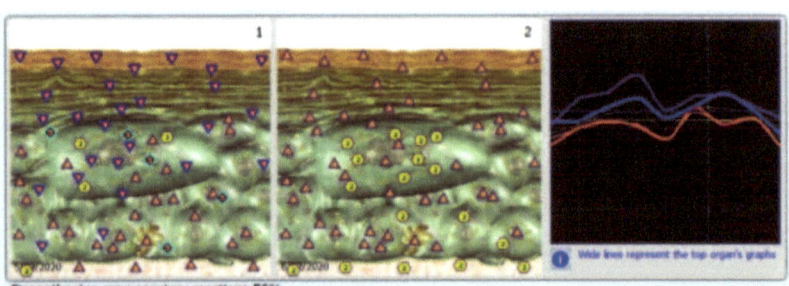
Strengthening compensatory reactions 56%
5/29/2020 Multilayer flat keratosic epithelium

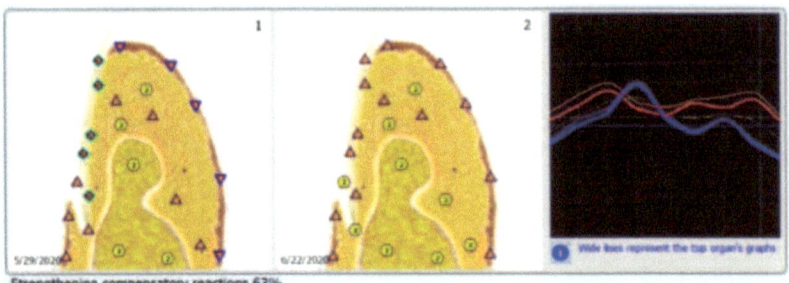
Strengthening compensatory reactions 63%
5/29/2020 Nail

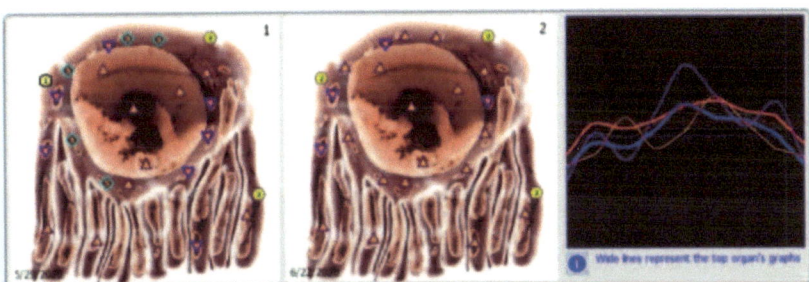

Strengthening compensatory reactions 45%
5/29/2020 Nephrocyte

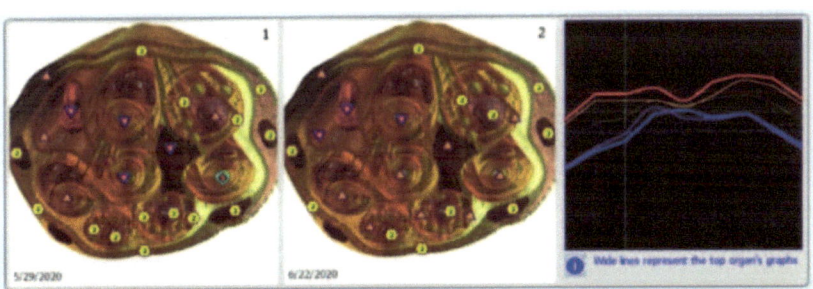

Strengthening compensatory reactions 13%
5/29/2020 Nerve bundle

Strengthening compensatory reactions 32%
5/29/2020 Nerves of maxilla and mandible:left view

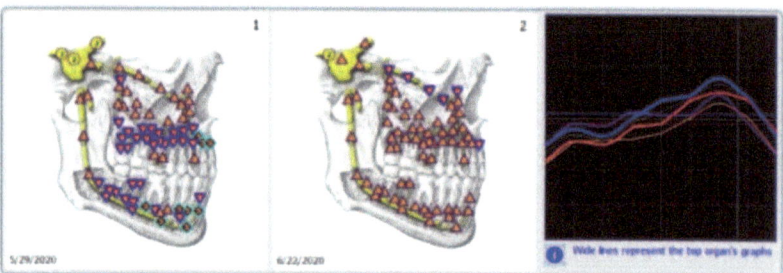

Strengthening compensatory reactions 46%

5/29/2020 Nerves of maxilla and mandible:right view

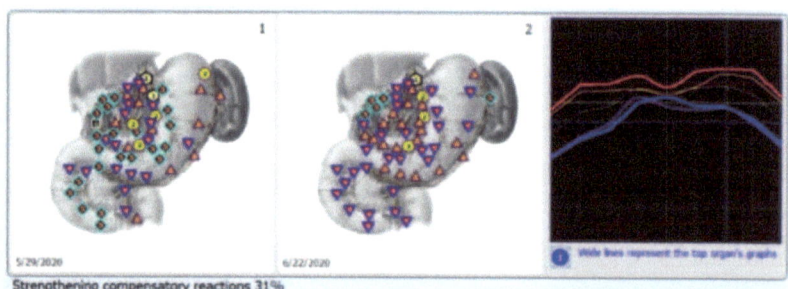

Strengthening compensatory reactions 31%
Decreasing of nidus of defeat by 100%
5/29/2020 Nerves of stomach

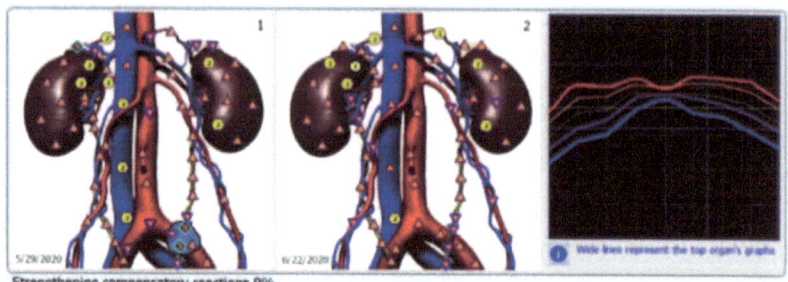

Strengthening compensatory reactions 9%

5/29/2020 Organs of retroperitoneal space

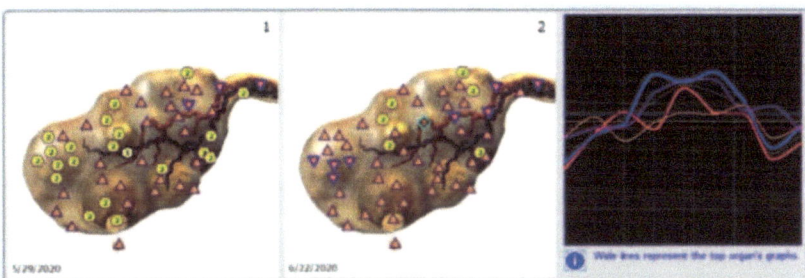
Weakening compensatory reactions 35%
5/29/2020 Ovary:right view

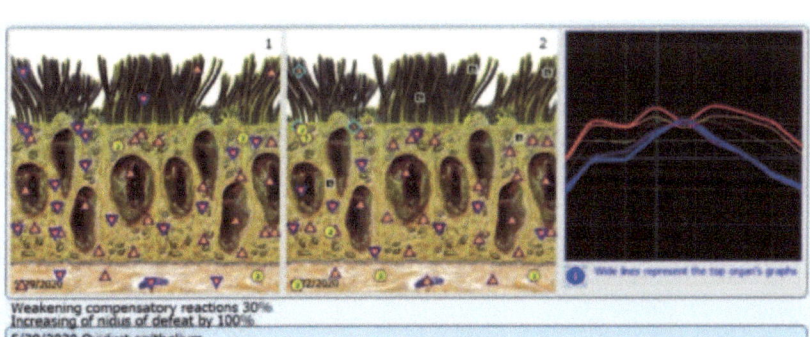
Weakening compensatory reactions 30%
Increasing of nidus of defeat by 100%
5/29/2020 Oviduct epithelium

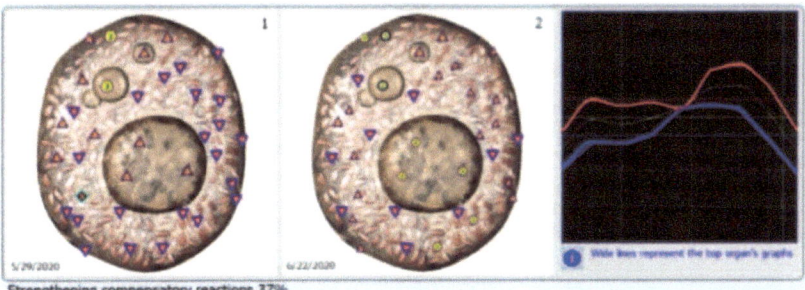
Strengthening compensatory reactions 37%
5/29/2020 Oxyphil cells of the parathyroid gland

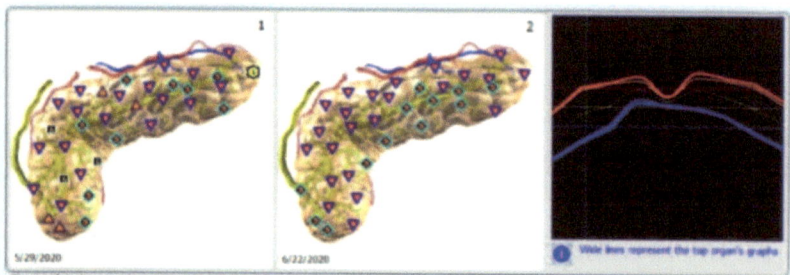

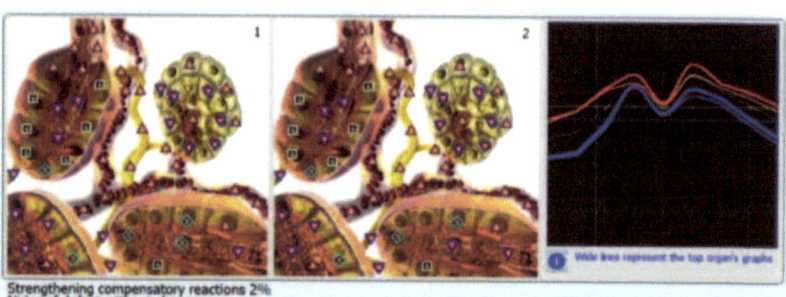

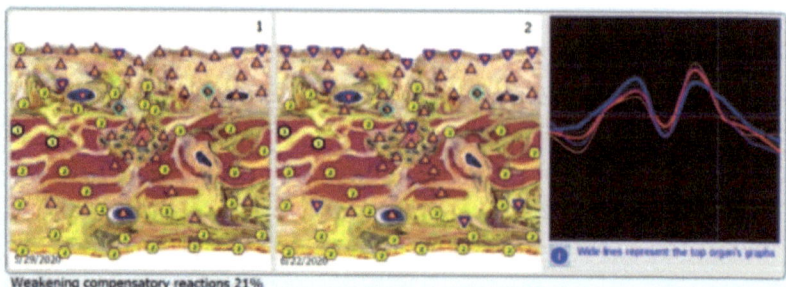

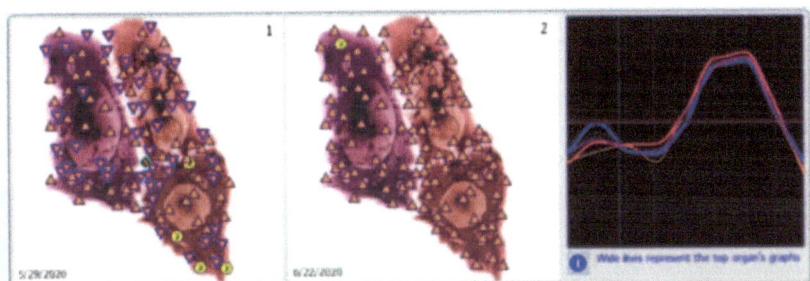
Strengthening compensatory reactions 39%
5/29/2020 Parathyrocyte

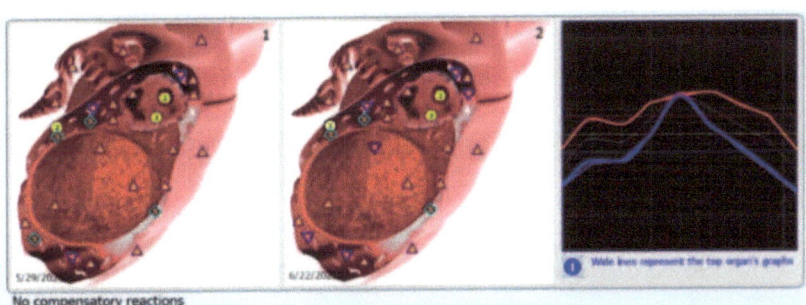
No compensatory reactions
5/29/2020 Podocyte

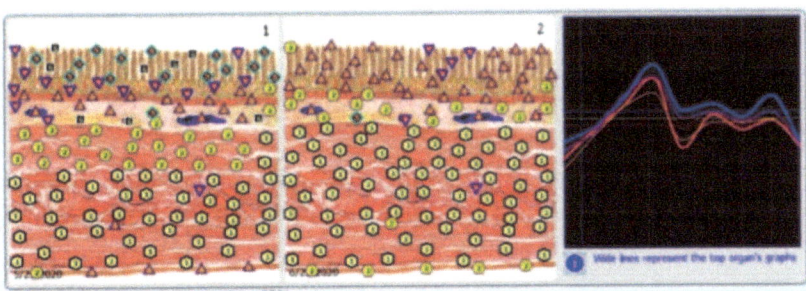
Strengthening compensatory reactions 69%
Decreasing of nidus of defeat by 100%
5/29/2020 Pyloric antrum

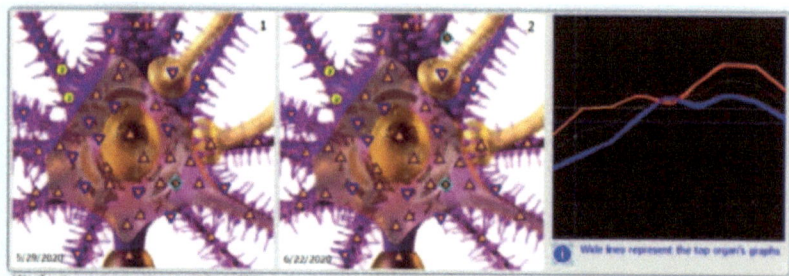

5/29/2020 Pyramidal neuron
Weakening compensatory reactions 1%

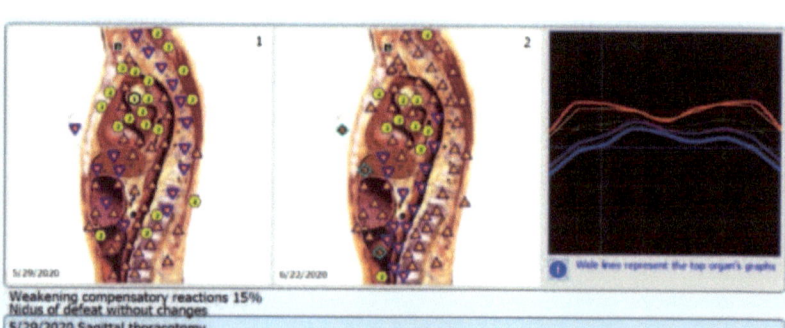

5/29/2020 Sagittal thoracotomy
Weakening compensatory reactions 15%
Nidus of defeat without changes

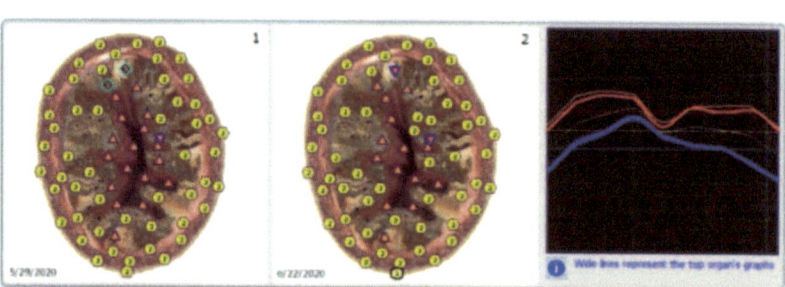

5/29/2020 Section of esophagus
Strengthening compensatory reactions 20%

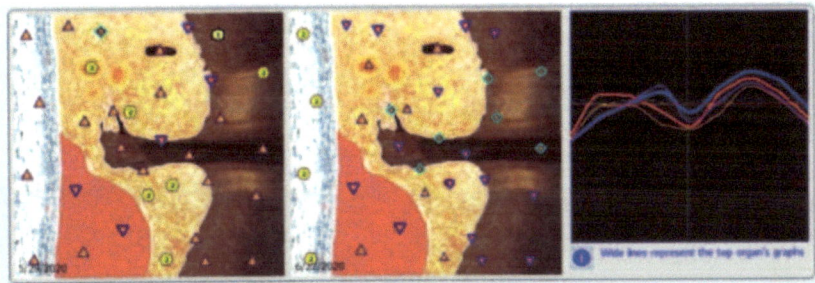

Weakening compensatory reactions 50%
5/29/2020 Section of larynx

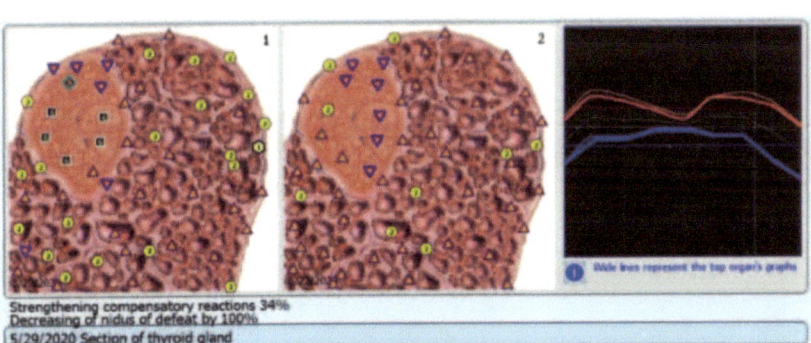

Strengthening compensatory reactions 34%
Decreasing of nidus of defeat by 100%
5/29/2020 Section of thyroid gland

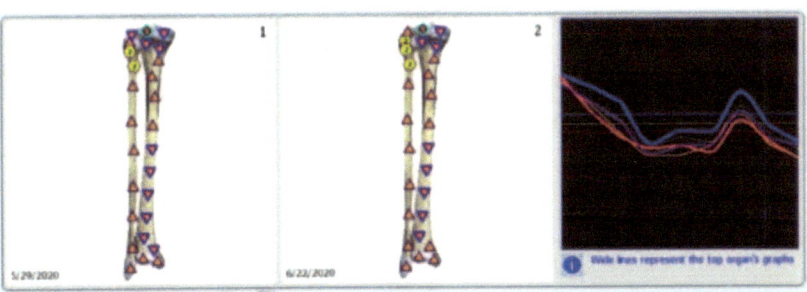

Strengthening compensatory reactions 8%
5/29/2020 Shin bones:left view

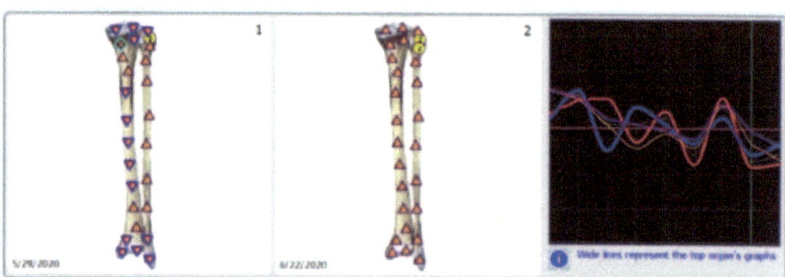

Strengthening compensatory reactions 48%
5/29/2020 Shin bones:right view

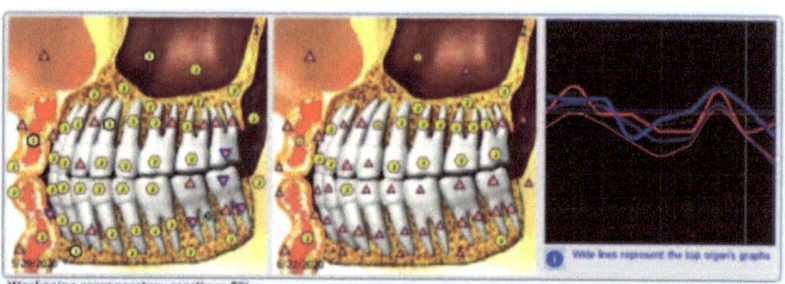

Weakening compensatory reactions 9%
5/29/2020 Teeth:left view

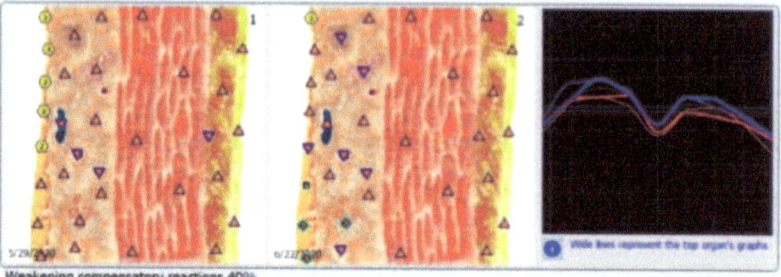

Weakening compensatory reactions 40%
Increasing of nidus of defeat by 100%
5/29/2020 Throat-sectional view

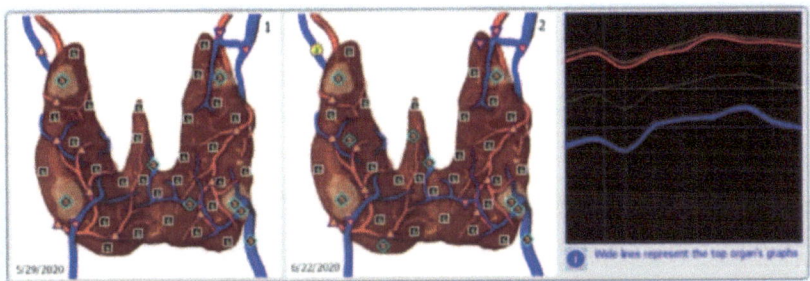

Strengthening compensatory reactions 7%
Decreasing of nidus of defeat by 14%
5/29/2020 Thyroid gland:from posterior view

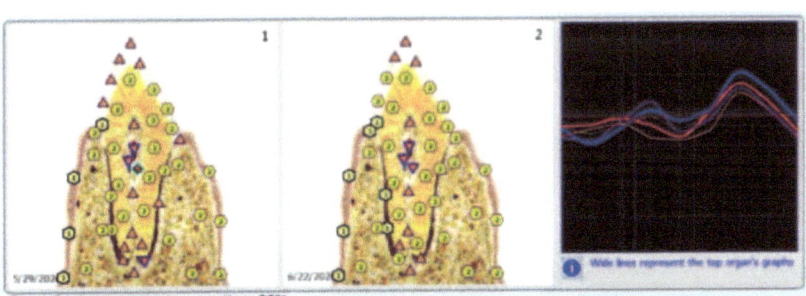

Strengthening compensatory reactions 26%
5/29/2020 Tooth

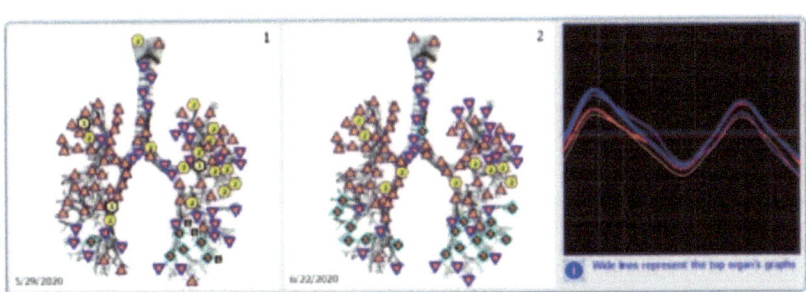

Weakening compensatory reactions 12%
Decreasing of nidus of defeat by 100%
5/29/2020 Trachea and bronchi

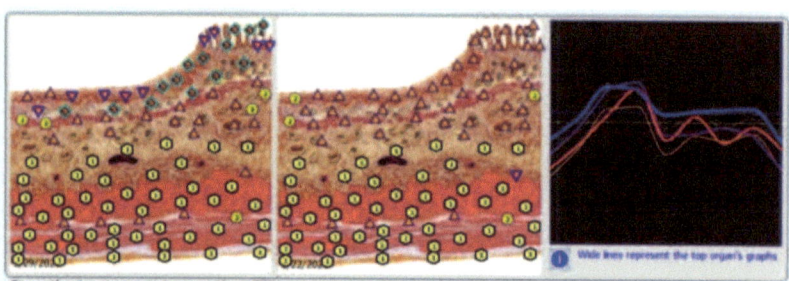

Strengthening compensatory reactions 55%
5/29/2020 Transition of esophagus to stomach

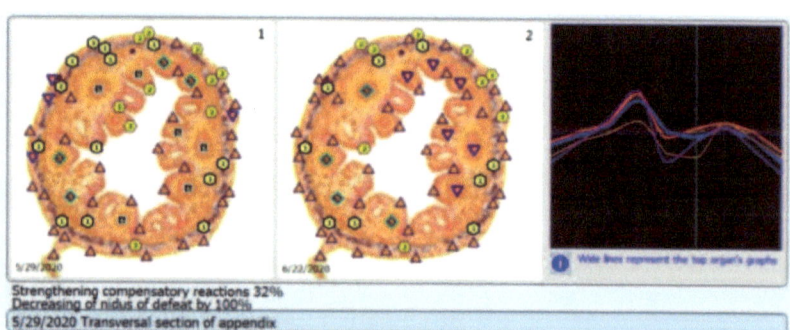

Strengthening compensatory reactions 32%
Decreasing of nidus of defeat by 100%
5/29/2020 Transversal section of appendix

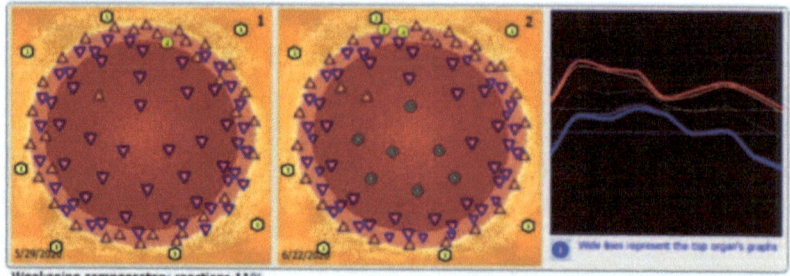

Weakening compensatory reactions 11%
5/29/2020 Transverse section of aorta

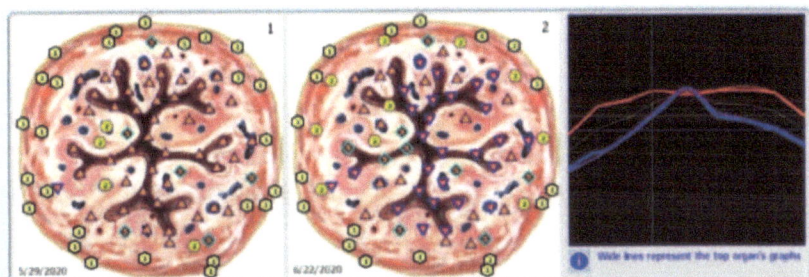
Weakening compensatory reactions 39%
5/29/2020 Urethra

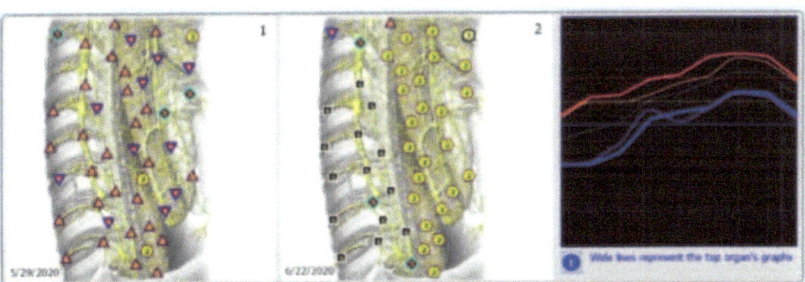
Weakening compensatory reactions 50%
Increasing of nidus of defeat by 100%
5/29/2020 Vegetative nervous system of abdomen:left view

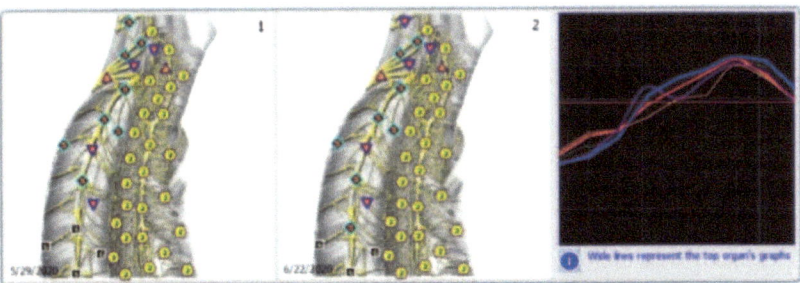
Strengthening compensatory reactions 6%
Decreasing of nidus of defeat by 25%
5/29/2020 Vegetative nervous system of thorax:left view

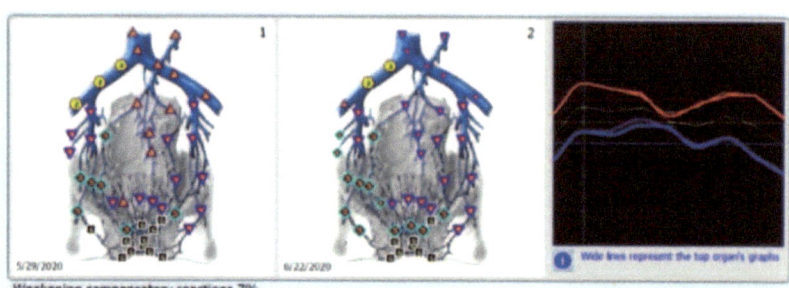

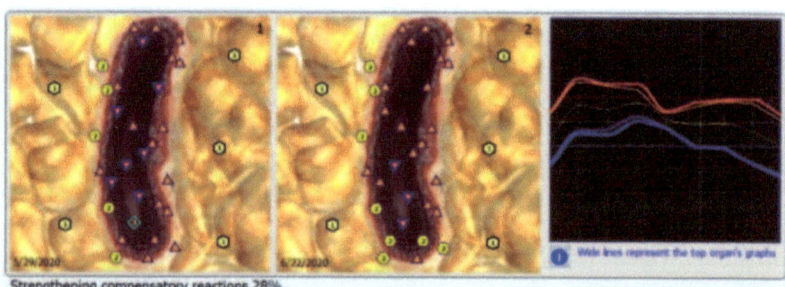

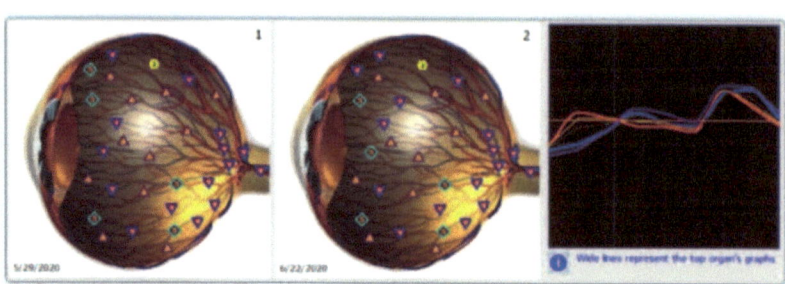

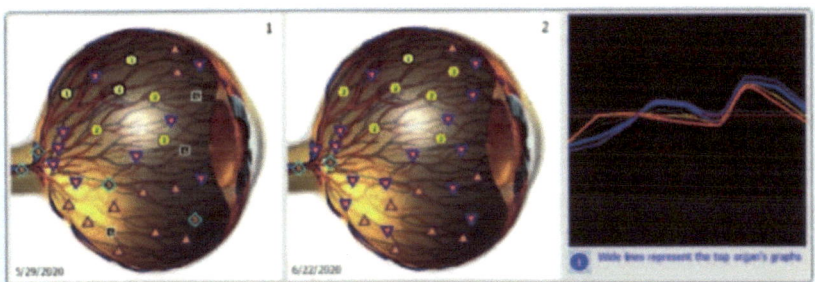

Strengthening compensatory reactions 27%
Decreasing of nidus of defeat by 100%
5/29/2020 Vessels of eye:right view

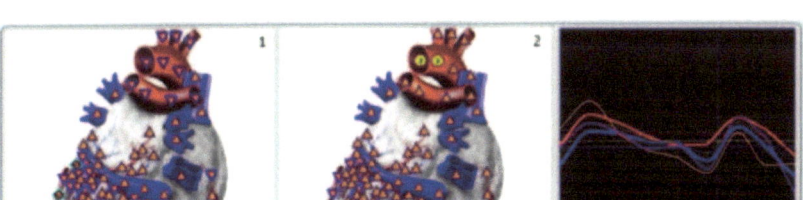

Strengthening compensatory reactions 40%
5/29/2020 Vessels of posterior heart wall

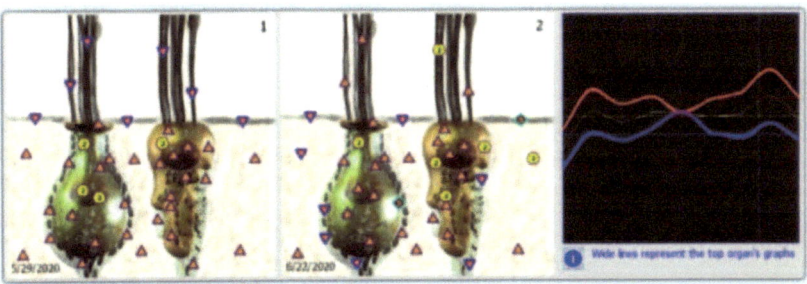

Weakening compensatory reactions 13%
5/29/2020 Vestibular cells

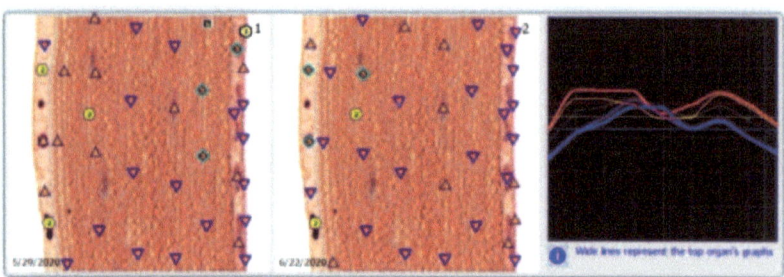

5/29/2020 Wall of aorta

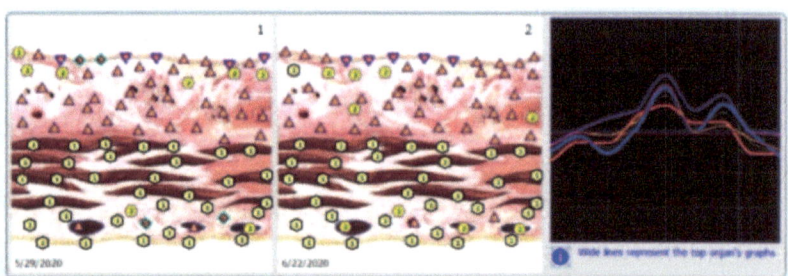

5/29/2020 Wall of cholic duct

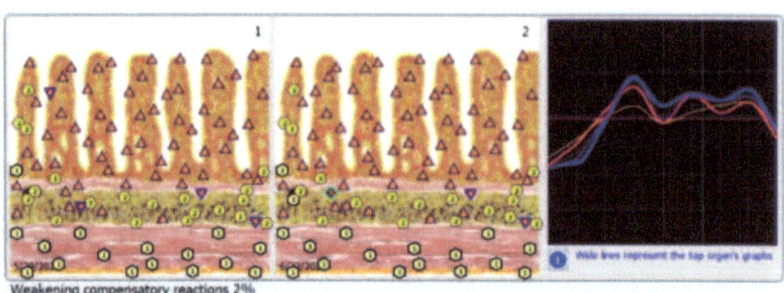

5/29/2020 Wall of doudenum

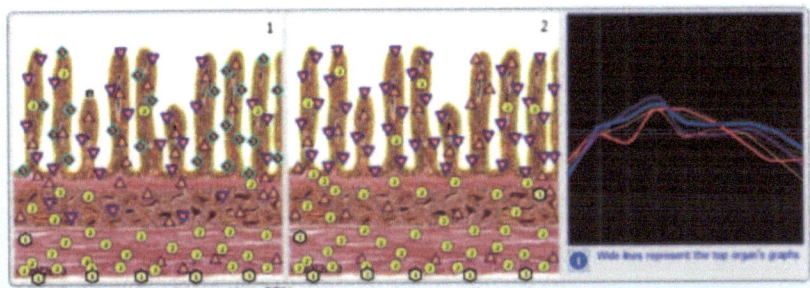

Strengthening compensatory reactions 35%
Decreasing of nidus of defeat by 100%
5/29/2020 Wall of small intestine

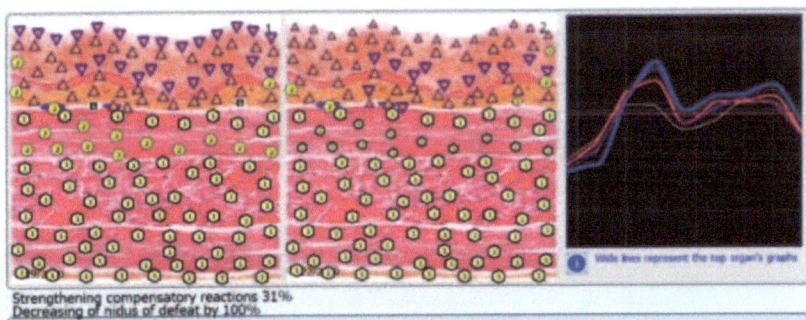

Strengthening compensatory reactions 31%
Decreasing of nidus of defeat by 100%
5/29/2020 Wall of stomach

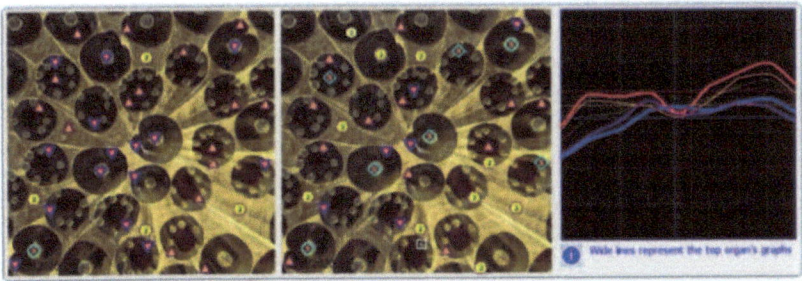

Weakening compensatory reactions 17%
Increasing of nidus of defeat by 100%
5/29/2020 White Matter

Magnetic Resonance Quantum Analyzer WF-QA46

Test Report 06/03/2020 vs 06/29/2020

https://qrgo.page.link/yD8QG

https://qrgo.page.link/2rMft

- Pancreatic function, slight increase of insulin level.

- Arterial Oxygen Content PaCO2, slight increase possible pathogen activity.

- Bone degeneration; adhesion degree of shoulder muscle from u.012 to u.0.14 (optimal is < u 0.2) slight worsening of aging of ligaments from 22% to 23%.

- Trace minerals; deficiency of potassium levels.

- Thyroid functions, FT4 slight increase.

- Toxin; mildly high levels of tobacco/nicotine.

- Heavy Metals; mildly high antimony levels.

- Pulse heart and brain; Stroke Volume (SV) from mildly deficient function to optimal values. Pulse wave coefficient K from normal values to mild deficiency.

18D Metatron NLS

Test Report 05/29/2020 vs 06/29/2020

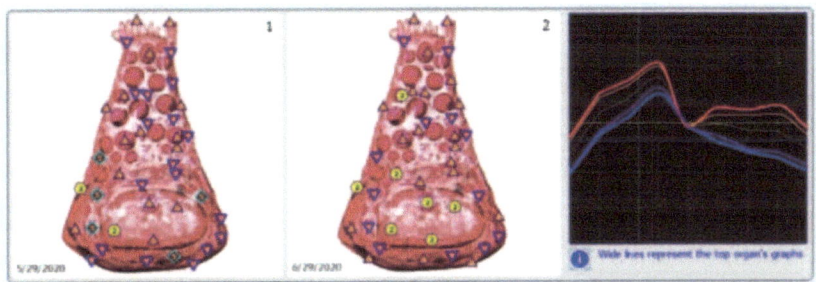

Strengthening compensatory reactions 35%
5/29/2020 Acinic insular cells of pancreas

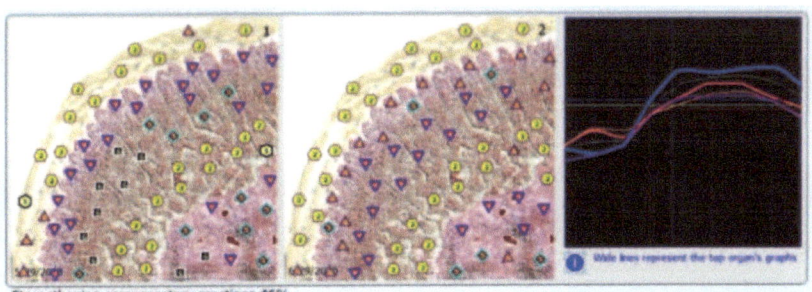

Strengthening compensatory reactions 46%
Decreasing of nidus of defeat by 100%
5/29/2020 Adrenal

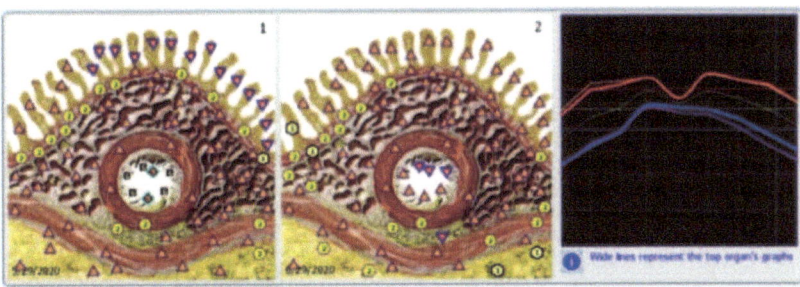

Strengthening compensatory reactions 42%
Decreasing of nidus of defeat by 100%
5/29/2020 Ampulla of vater duct

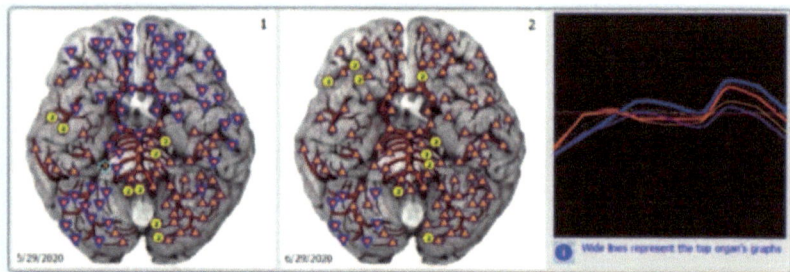

Strengthening compensatory reactions 39%
5/29/2020 Arteries of brain:view from below

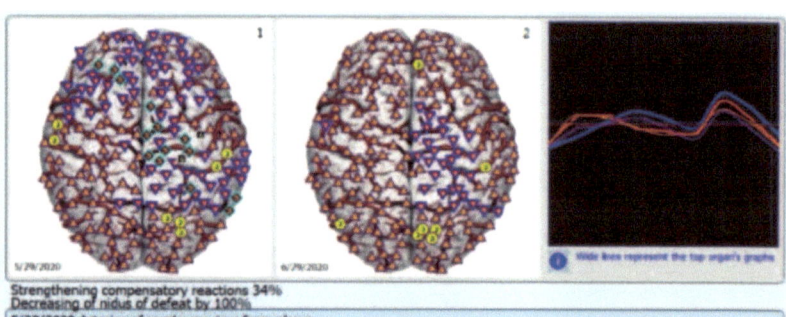

Strengthening compensatory reactions 34%
Decreasing of nidus of defeat by 100%
5/29/2020 Arteries of cerebrum:view from above

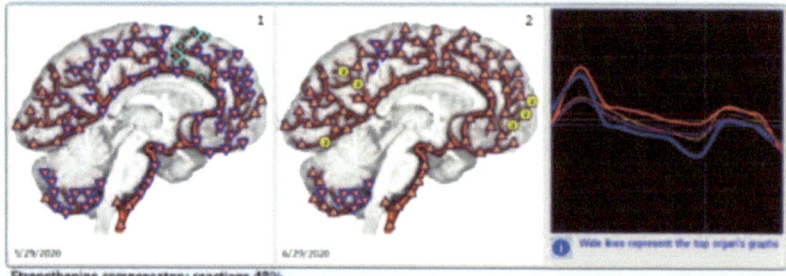

Strengthening compensatory reactions 48%
5/29/2020 Arteries of the medial surface of cerebrum:left view

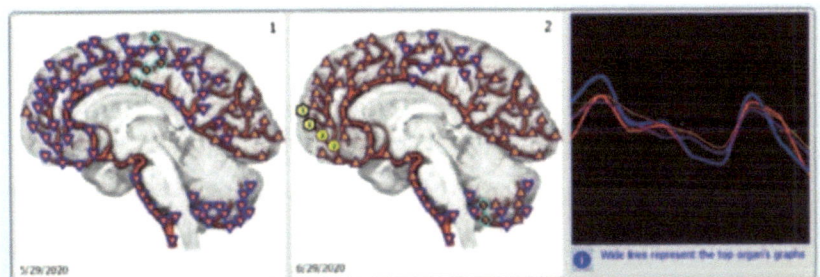
Strengthening compensatory reactions 40%
5/29/2020 Arteries of the medial surface of cerebrum:right view

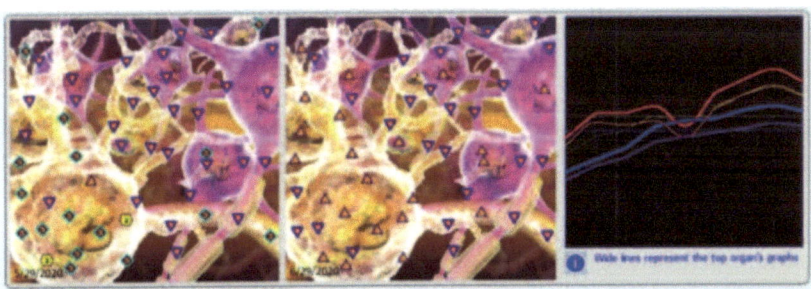
Strengthening compensatory reactions 41%
5/29/2020 Astrocytes

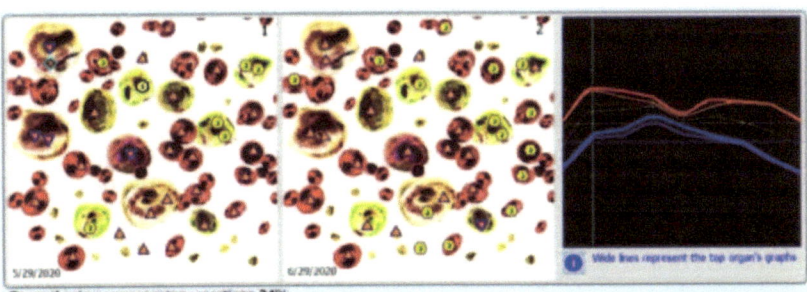
Strengthening compensatory reactions 34%
5/29/2020 Blood cells

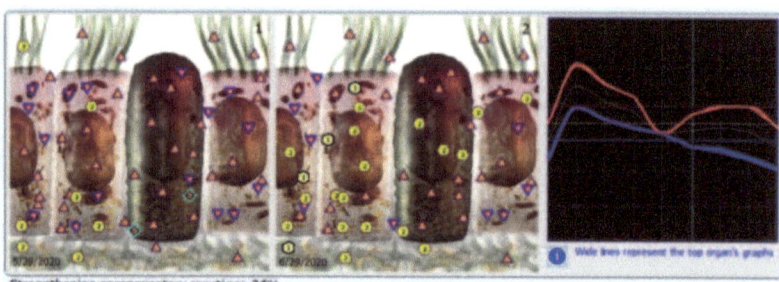
Strengthening compensatory reactions 34%
5/29/2020 Bronchiolar epithelium

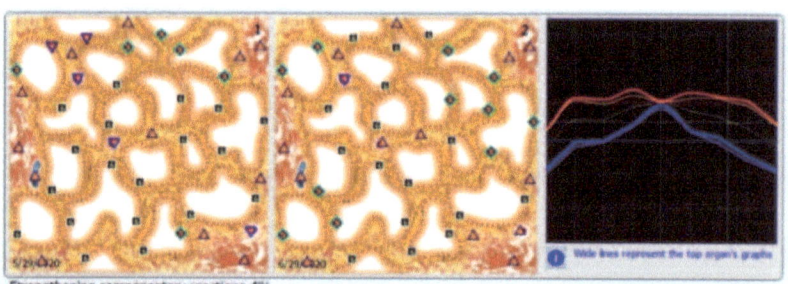
Strengthening compensatory reactions 4%
Decreasing of nidus of defeat by 16%
5/29/2020 Bulbourethral glands

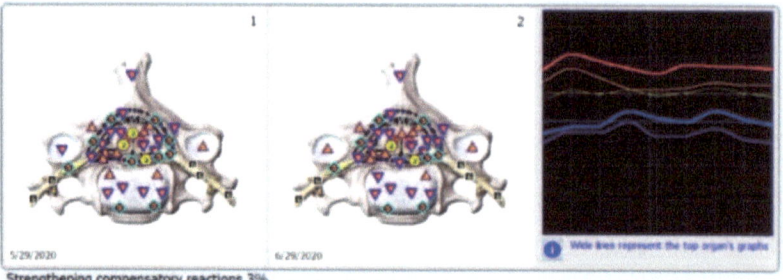
Strengthening compensatory reactions 3%
Nidus of defeat without changes
5/29/2020 Fourth neck-bone

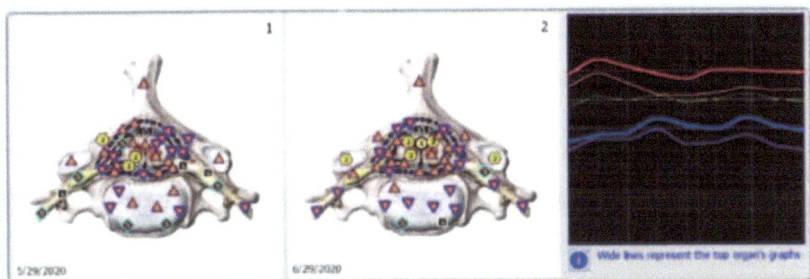

Strengthening compensatory reactions 27%
Decreasing of nidus of defeat by 67%
5/29/2020 Fifth neck-bone

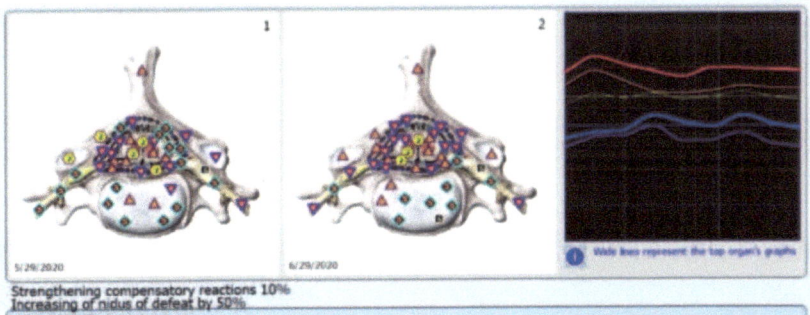

Strengthening compensatory reactions 10%
Increasing of nidus of defeat by 50%
5/29/2020 Sixth neck-bone

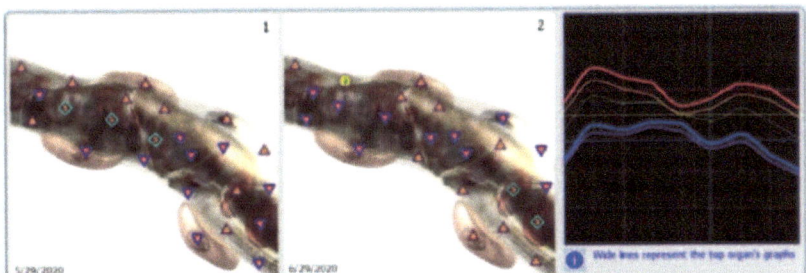

Strengthening compensatory reactions 9%
5/29/2020 Capillar

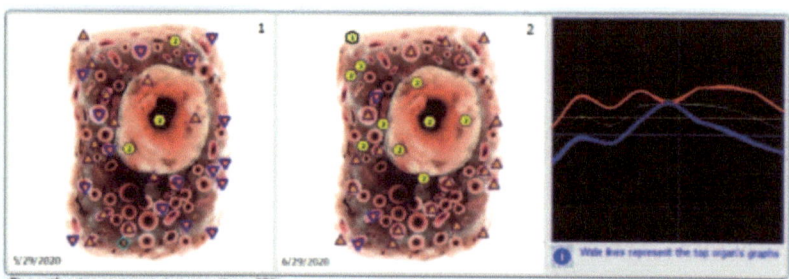
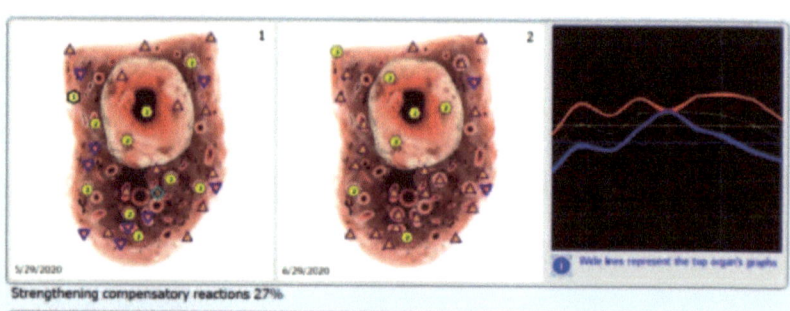
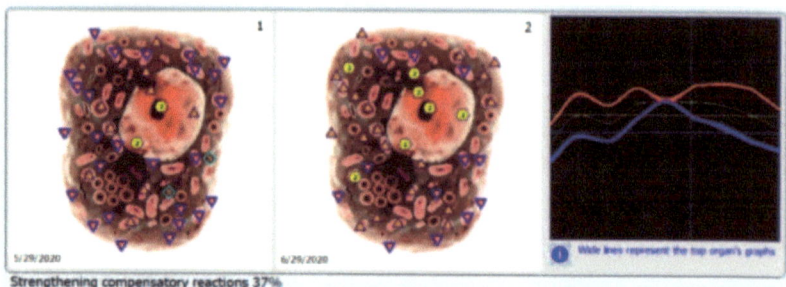

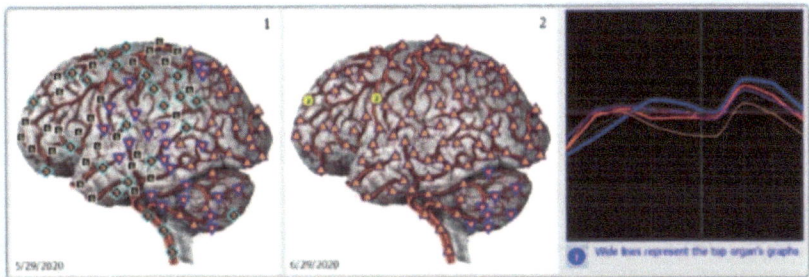

Strengthening compensatory reactions 74%
Decreasing of nidus of defeat by 100%
5/29/2020 Cerebral arteries:lateral view of left hemisphere

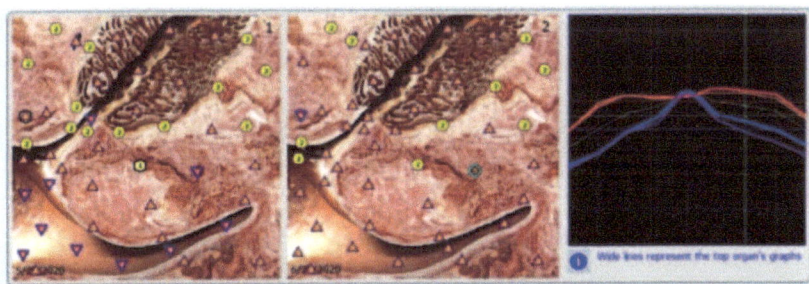

Strengthening compensatory reactions 10%
5/29/2020 Cervix uteri(neck of uterus)

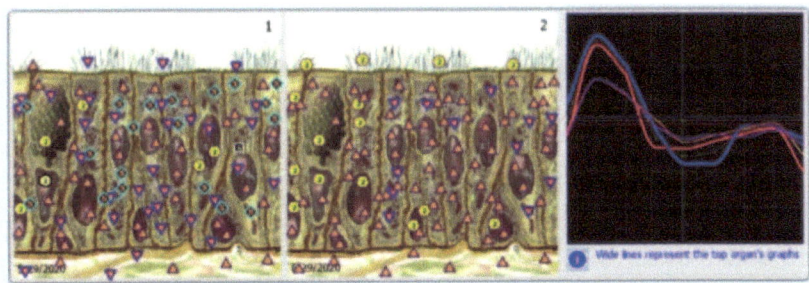

Strengthening compensatory reactions 52%
Decreasing of nidus of defeat by 100%
5/29/2020 Ciliated epithelial cell

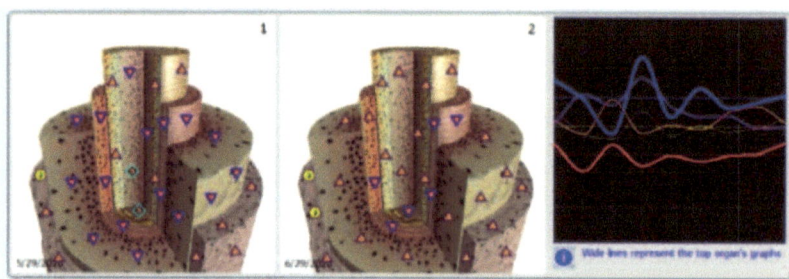

Strengthening compensatory reactions 37%
5/29/2020 Cuticle of hair

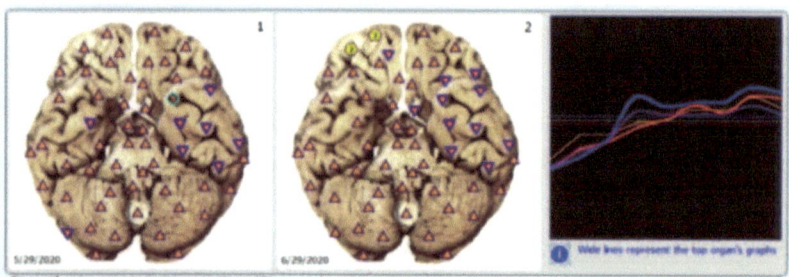

Strengthening compensatory reactions 1%
5/29/2020 Encephalon,cranial nerves: bottom view

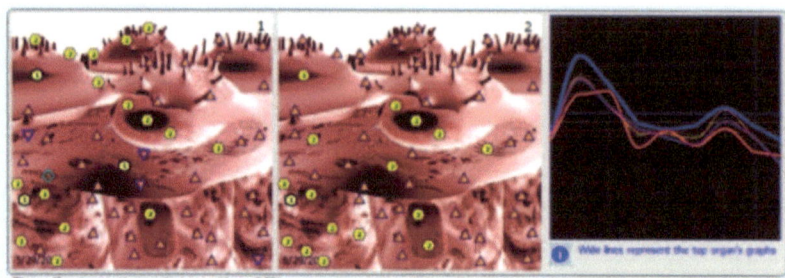

Strengthening compensatory reactions 14%
5/29/2020 Endothelial cells

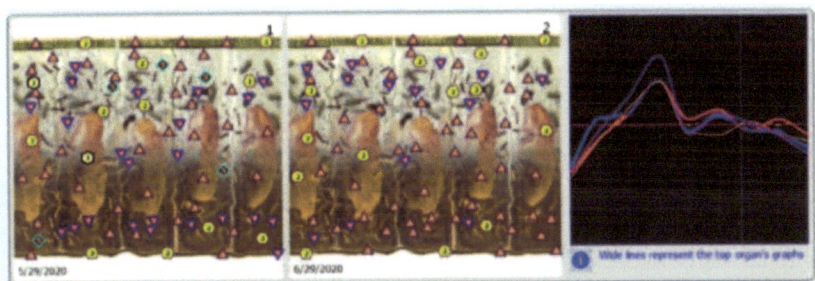

Strengthening compensatory reactions 26%

5/29/2020 Epithelial cell of intestine

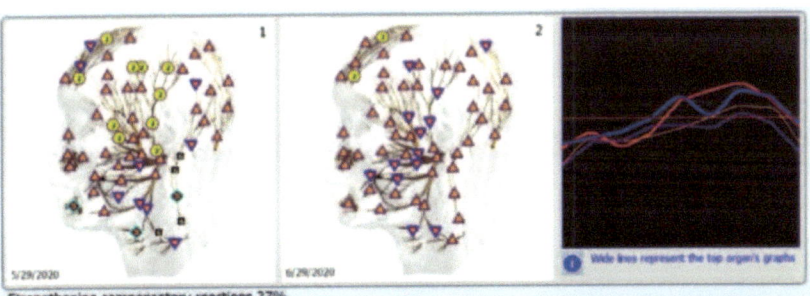

Strengthening compensatory reactions 27%
Decreasing of nidus of defeat by 100%

5/29/2020 Facial nerve:left view

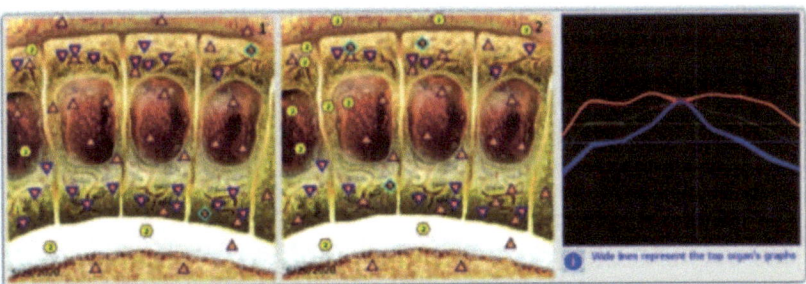

Strengthening compensatory reactions 13%

5/29/2020 Follicular ovary cells

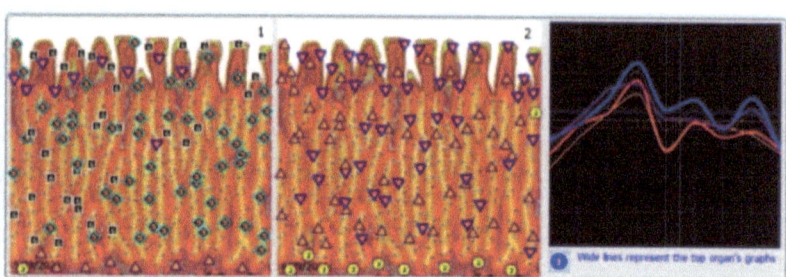

Strengthening compensatory reactions 71%
Decreasing of nidus of defeat by 100%
5/29/2020 Gastric glands

Strengthening compensatory reactions 56%
Decreasing of nidus of defeat by 100%
5/29/2020 Gray matter of cerebrum

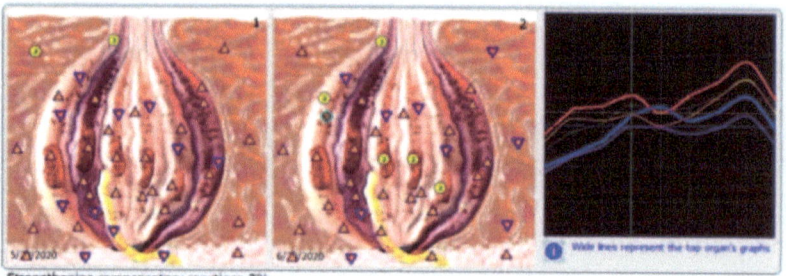

Strengthening compensatory reactions 2%
5/29/2020 Gustatory bud

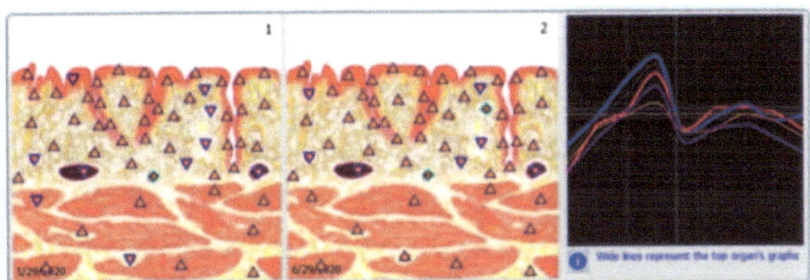
Strengthening compensatory reactions 1%
5/29/2020 Lingual papilla

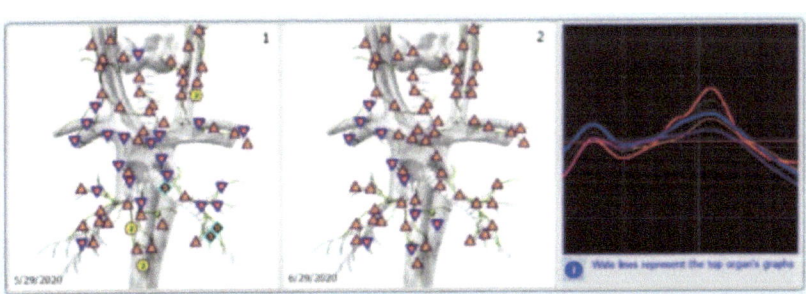
Strengthening compensatory reactions 22%
5/29/2020 Lymphatic vessels of mediastinum

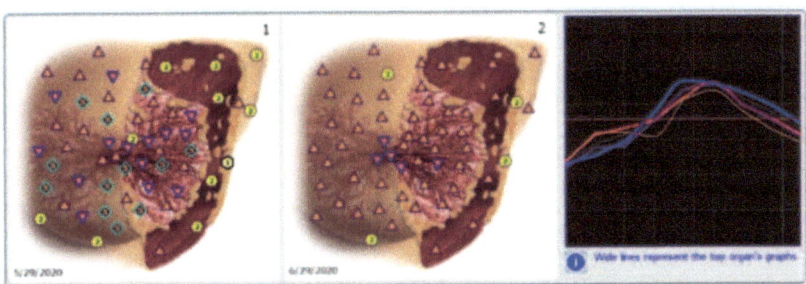
Strengthening compensatory reactions 45%
5/29/2020 Mammary gland duct:left view

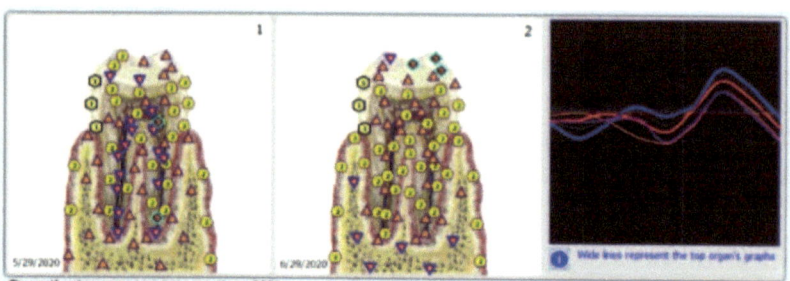

Strengthening compensatory reactions 19%
5/29/2020 Molar tooth

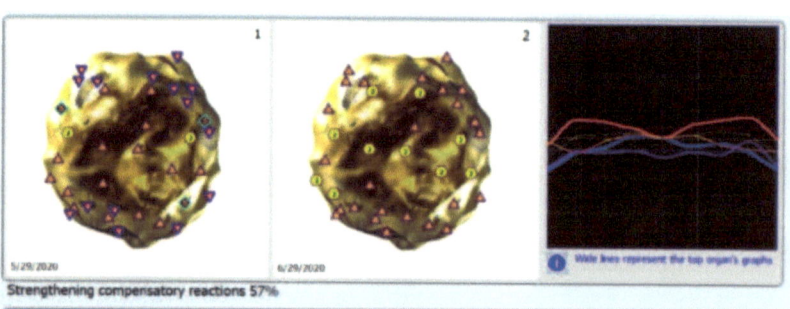

Strengthening compensatory reactions 57%
5/29/2020 Monocyte

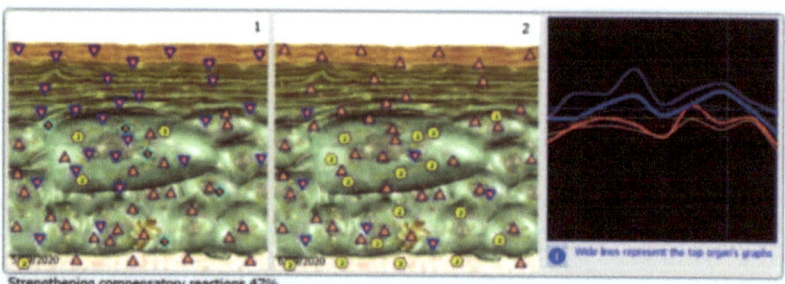

Strengthening compensatory reactions 47%
5/29/2020 Multilayer flat keratosic epithelium

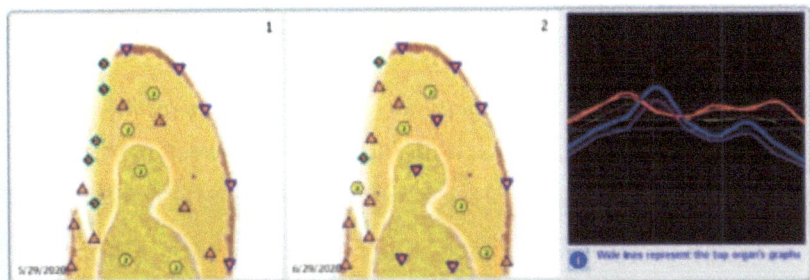
Strengthening compensatory reactions 15%
5/29/2020 Nail

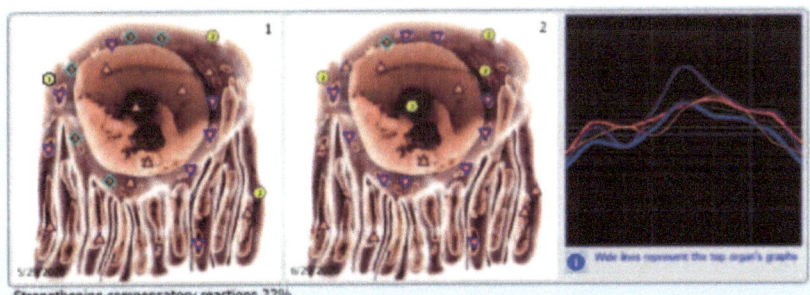
Strengthening compensatory reactions 22%
5/29/2020 Nephrocyte

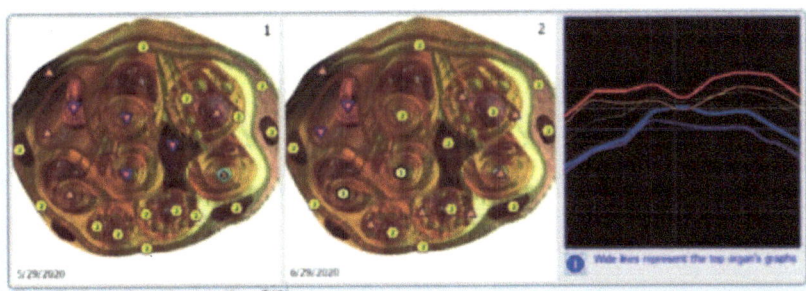
Strengthening compensatory reactions 31%
5/29/2020 Nerve bundle

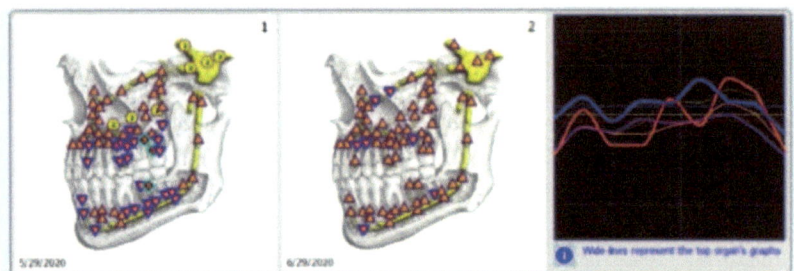

Strengthening compensatory reactions 27%
5/29/2020 Nerves of maxilla and mandible:left view

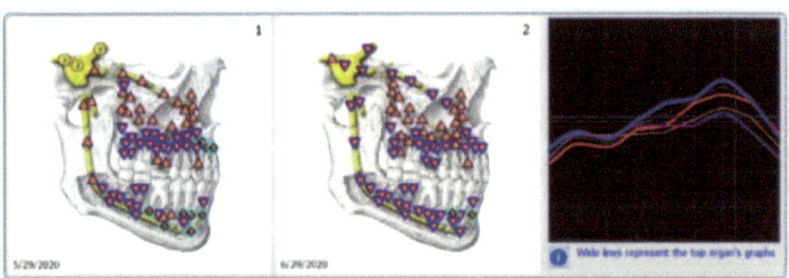

Strengthening compensatory reactions 4%
5/29/2020 Nerves of maxilla and mandible:right view

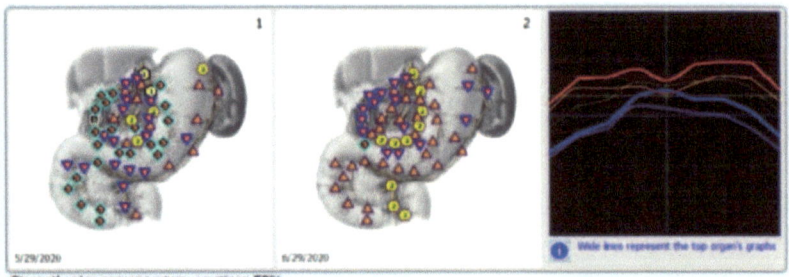

Strengthening compensatory reactions 53%
Decreasing of nidus of defeat by 100%
5/29/2020 Nerves of stomach

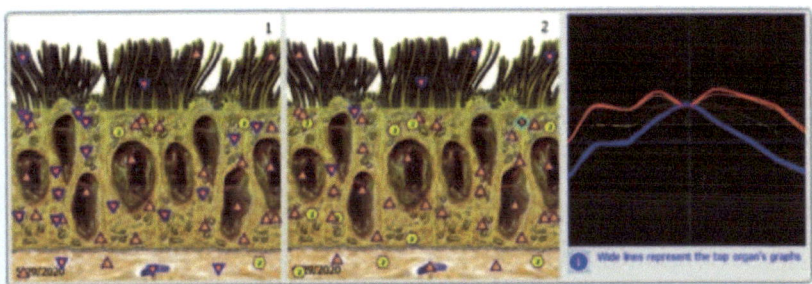
Strengthening compensatory reactions 29%
5/29/2020 Oviduct epithelium

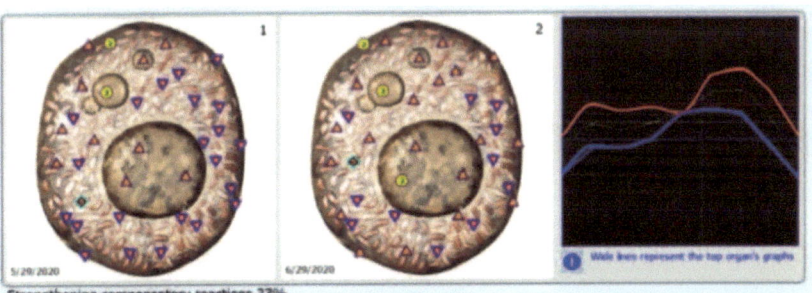
Strengthening compensatory reactions 23%
5/29/2020 Oxyphil cells of the parathyroid gland

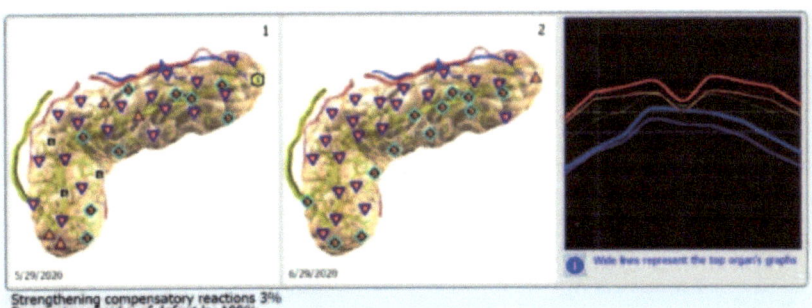
Strengthening compensatory reactions 3%
Decreasing of nidus of defeat by 100%
5/29/2020 Pancreas:front view

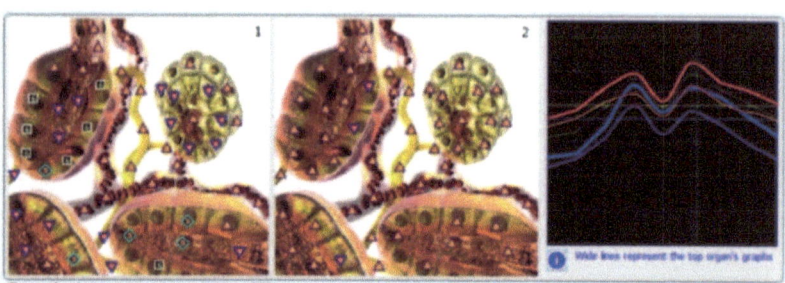

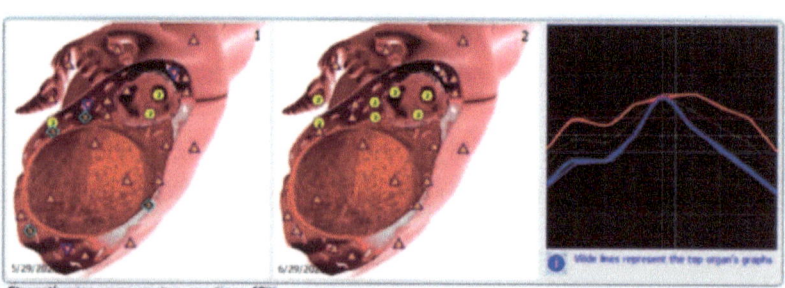

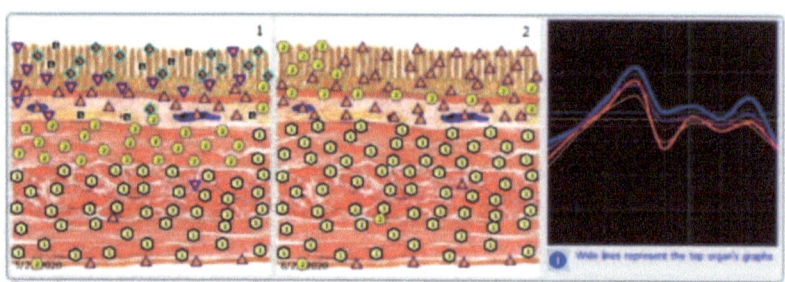

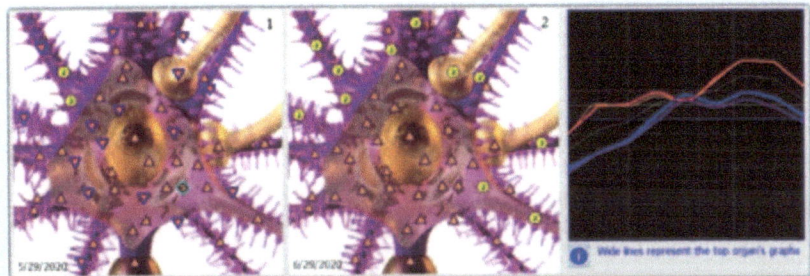

Strengthening compensatory reactions 45%

5/29/2020 Pyramidal neuron

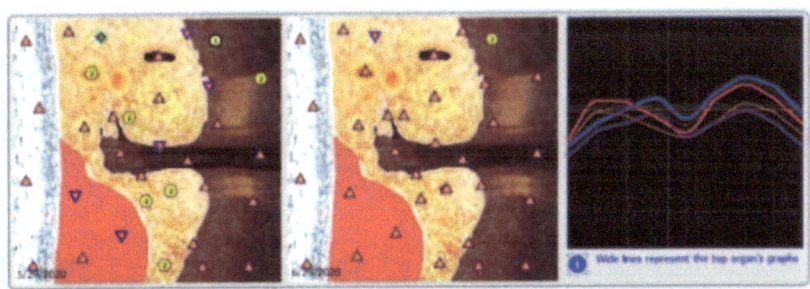

Strengthening compensatory reactions 12%

5/29/2020 Section of larynx

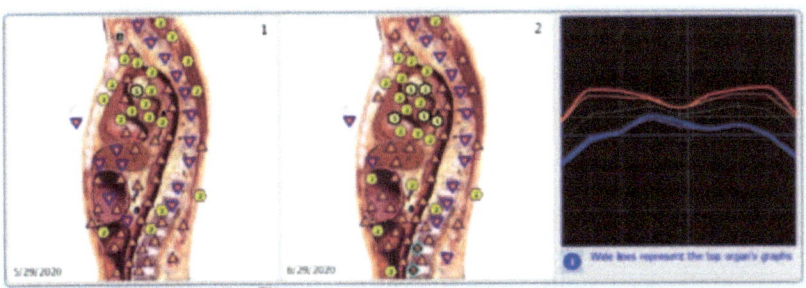

Strengthening compensatory reactions 7%
Decreasing of nidus of defeat by 100%

5/29/2020 Sagittal thoracotomy

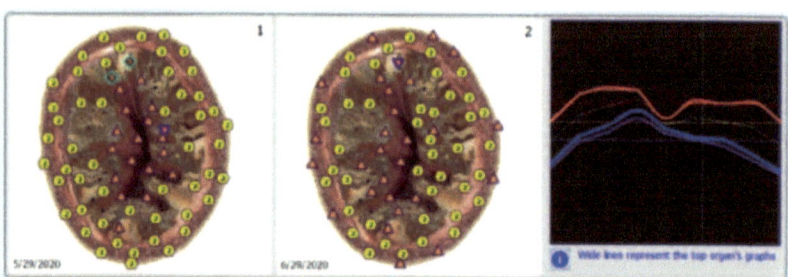
5/29/2020 Section of esophagus

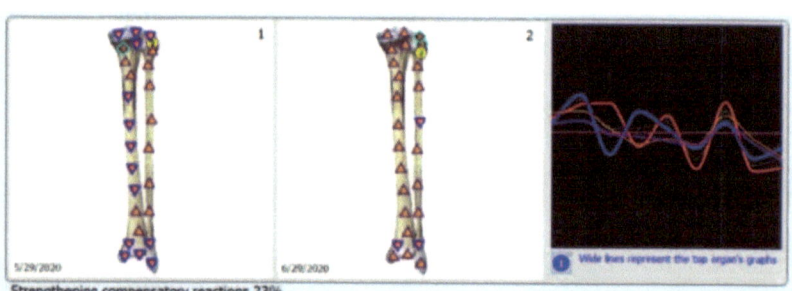
5/29/2020 Shin bones:right view

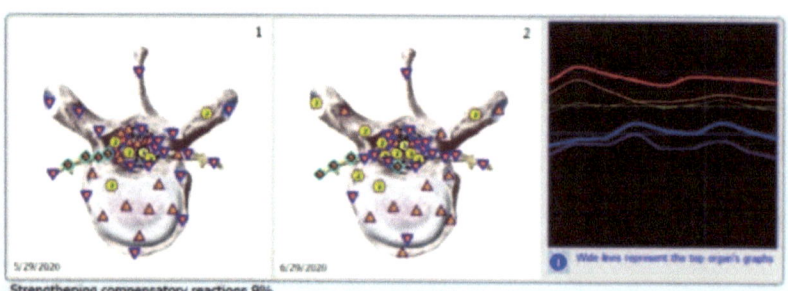
5/29/2020 First thoracic vertebra

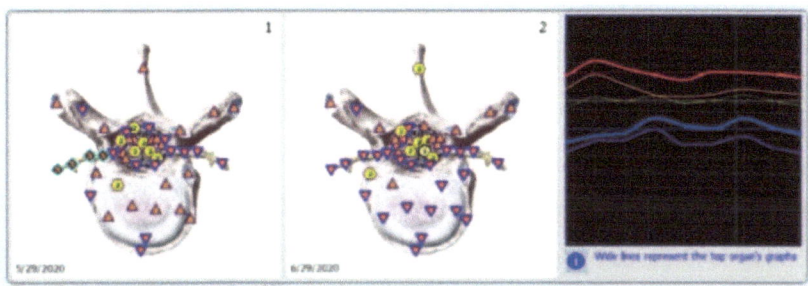

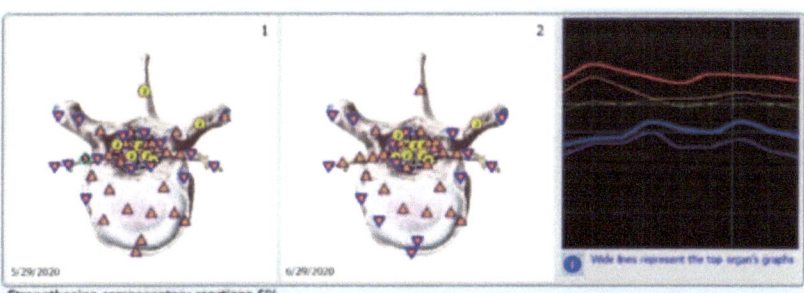

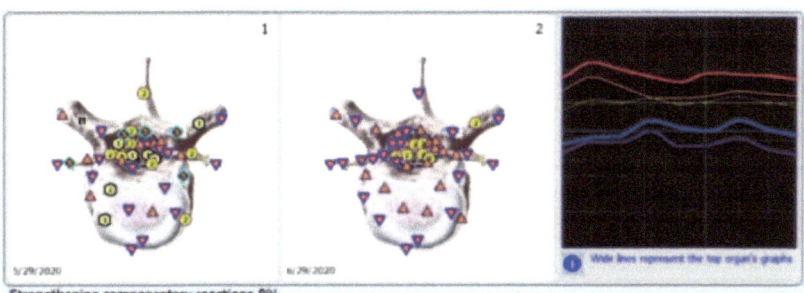

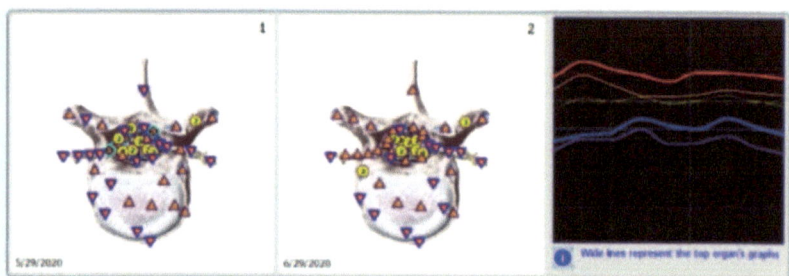

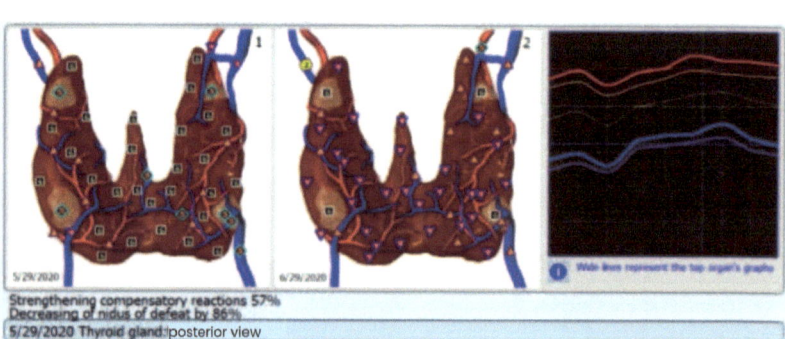

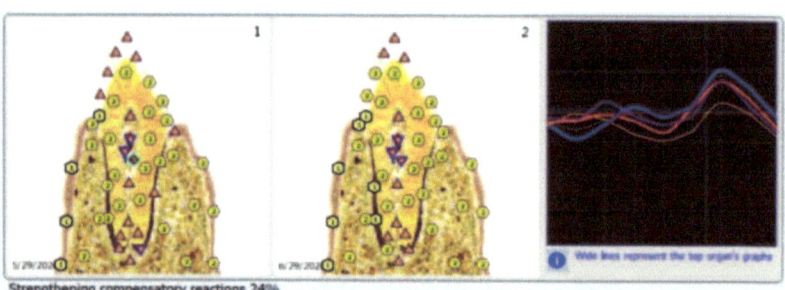

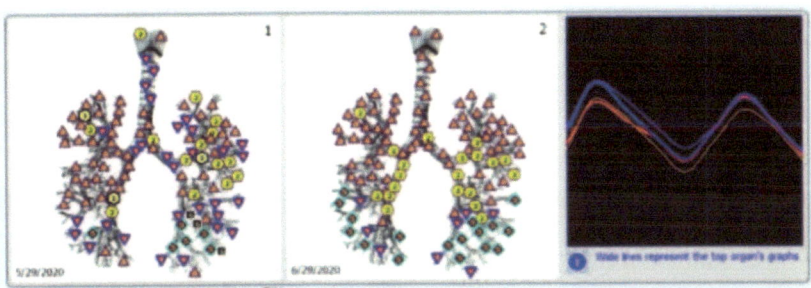

Strengthening compensatory reactions 7%
Decreasing of nidus of defeat by 100%
5/29/2020 Trachea and bronchi

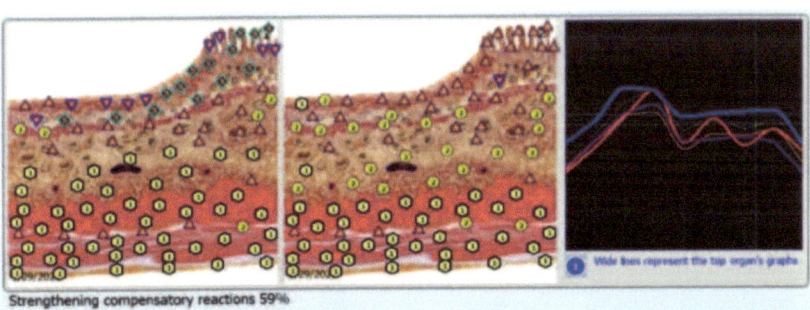

Strengthening compensatory reactions 59%
5/29/2020 Transition of esophagus to stomach

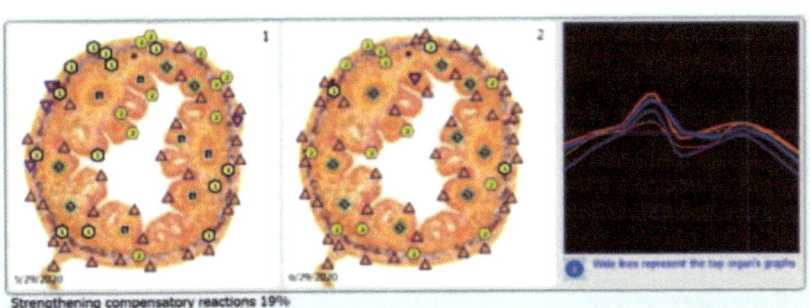

Strengthening compensatory reactions 19%
Decreasing of nidus of defeat by 100%
5/29/2020 Transversal section of appendix

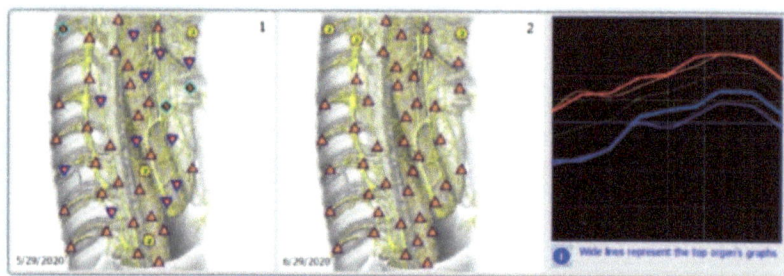
Strengthening compensatory reactions 38%
5/29/2020 Vegetative nervous system of abdomen:left view

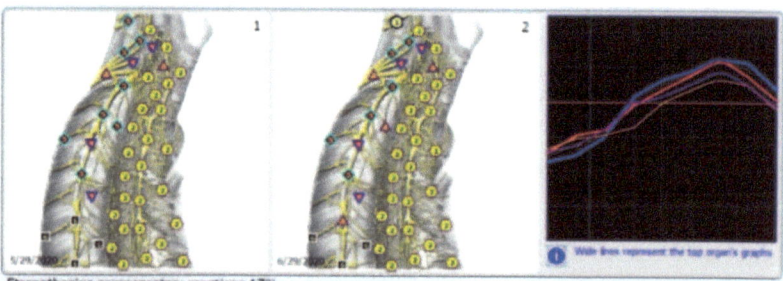
Strengthening compensatory reactions 17%
Decreasing of nidus of defeat by 25%
5/29/2020 Vegetative nervous system of thorax:left view

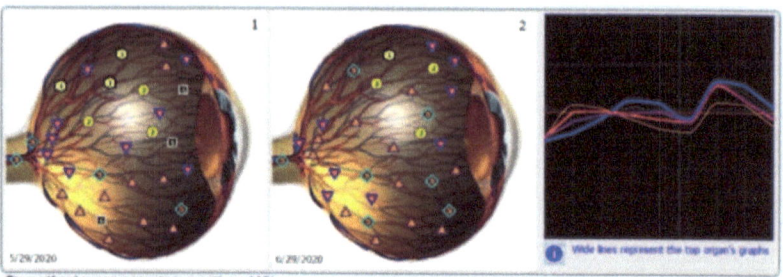
Strengthening compensatory reactions 11%
Decreasing of nidus of defeat by 100%
5/29/2020 Vessels of eye:right view

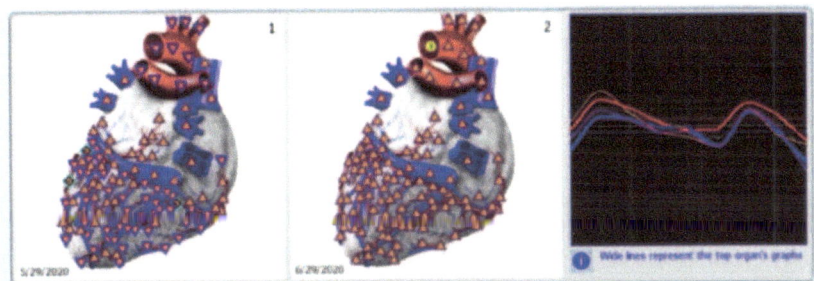
Strengthening compensatory reactions 45%
5/29/2020 Vessels of posterior heart wall

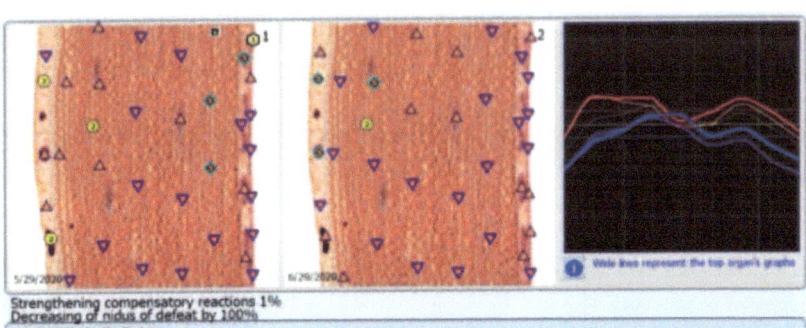
Strengthening compensatory reactions 1%
Decreasing of nidus of defeat by 100%
5/29/2020 Wall of aorta

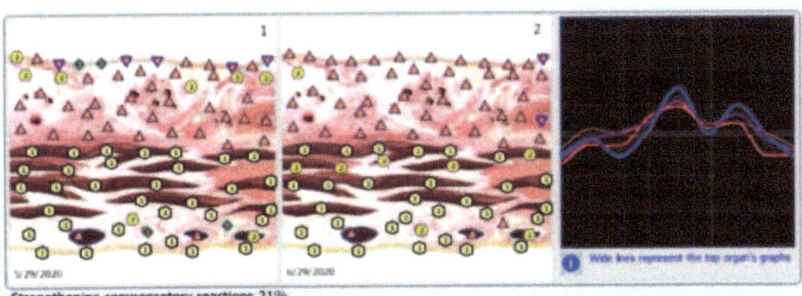
Strengthening compensatory reactions 21%
5/29/2020 Wall of cholic duct

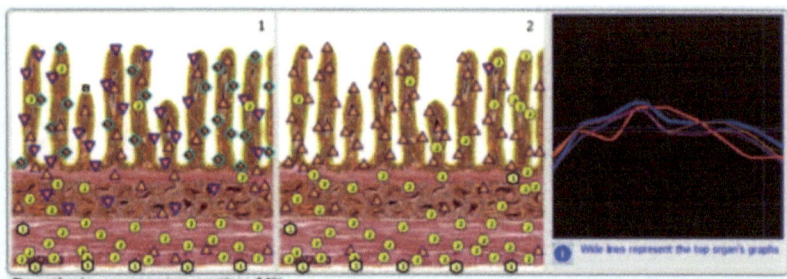

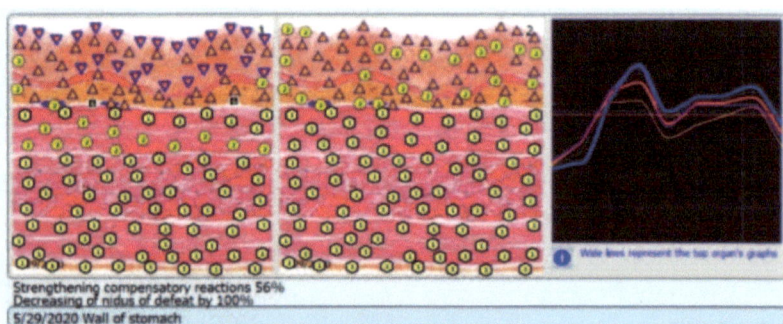

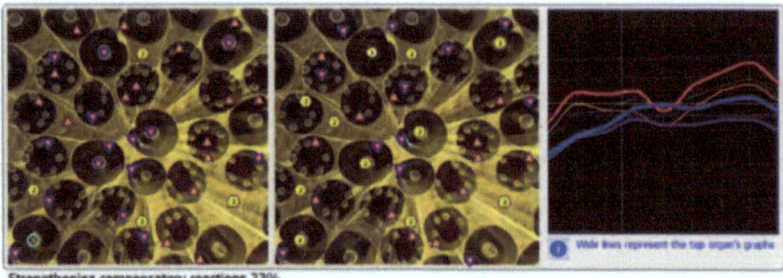

Before/After
Tx$_0$ vs Tx$_3$ on 06/29/2020

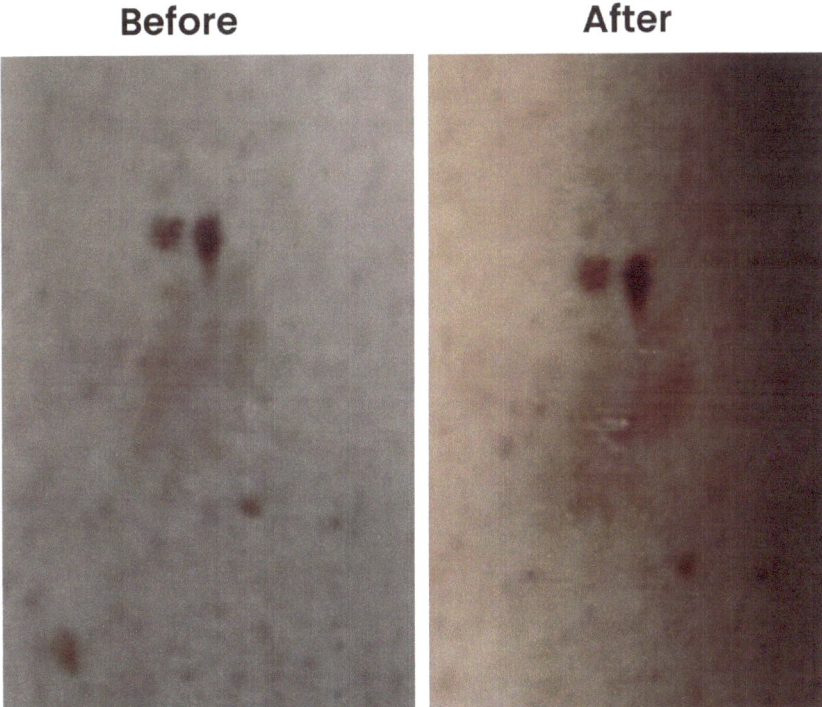

Before · After

Before/After
Tx$_0$ vs Tx$_3$ on 06/29/2020

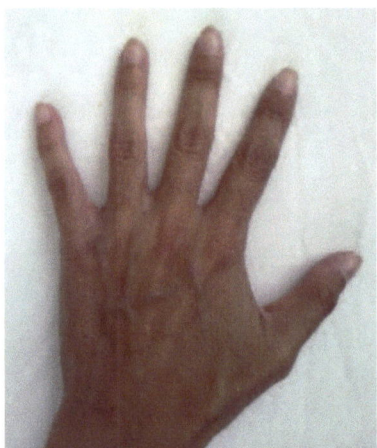

Before

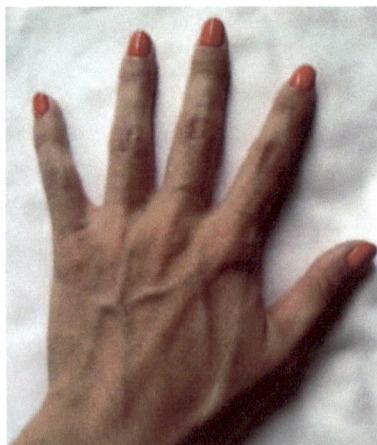

After

Before/After
Tx$_0$ vs Tx$_3$ on 06/29/2020

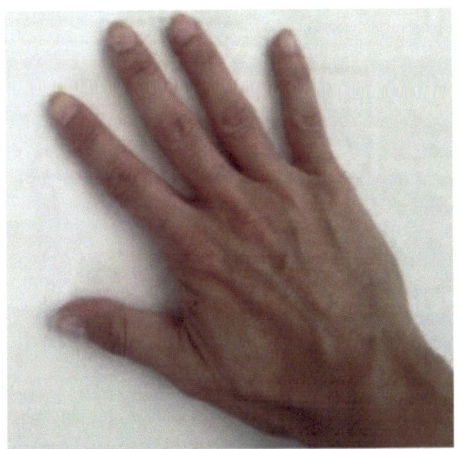

Before

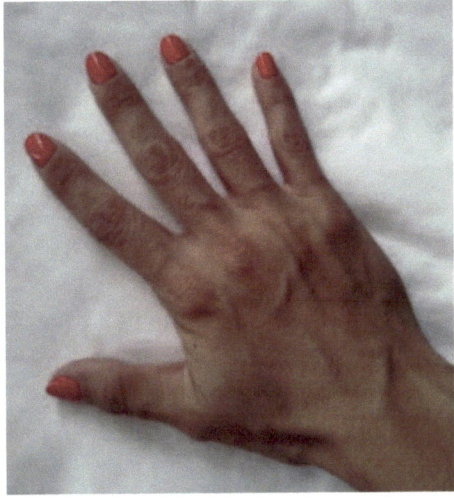

After

CONCLUSION

Overall, the health evaluation shows an enhancement of the core processes and strengthened compensatory response.

The scar edges are smoothened, scar size reduced, and skin complexion more even. A superficial exfoliation can be observed on the scarred area, possibly leading to an ongoing cellular turnover for at least two more weeks after the therapy.

Reduction of TEWL and restored proteins in the ECM are associated with more radiant and elastic tissue.
A moderate reduction of hands glycation is immediately noticeable at the snuff box, extensor tendons and phalangeal joints areas.

Highlighted a significant change from dull to a more radiant and healthier skin, increase in firmness associated with improved skin elasticity of hands.

BIBLIOGRAPHY

Bland, J. S. **(2014)**. *The disease delusion: Conquering the causes of chronic illness for a healthier, longer, and happier life.* HarperCollins.

Brinker, F. **(2010)**. *Herbal contraindications and drug interactions: Plus herbal adjuncts with medicines* (4th ed.).

Burlando, B., Verotta, L., Cornara, L., & Bottini-Massa, E. **(2010)**. *Herbal principles in cosmetics: Properties and mechanisms of action.* CRC Press.

Busia, K. **(2016)**. *Fundamentals of herbal medicine: History, Phytopharmacology and Phytotherapeutics.* Xlibris Corporation.

Busia, K. **(2016)**. *Fundamentals of herbal medicine: Major plant families, analytical methods, materia medica.* Xlibris Corporation.

Hibbott, H. W. **(2016)**. *Handbook of cosmetic science: An introduction to principles and applications.* Elsevier.

Lobo, V., Patil, A., Phatak, A., & Chandra, N. **(2010)**. *Free radicals, antioxidants and functional foods: Impact on human health.* Pharmacognosy Reviews, 4(8), 118. https://doi.org/10.4103/0973-7847.70902

Mehrandish, R., Rahimian, A., & Shahriary, A. **(2019)**. *Heavy metals detoxification: A review of herbal compounds for chelation therapy in heavy metals toxicity.* Journal of Herbmed Pharmacology, 8(2), 69-77. https://doi.org/10.15171/jhp.2019.12

Pillai, S., Oresajo, C., & Hayward, J. **(2005)**. *Ultraviolet radiation and skin aging: Roles of reactive oxygen species, inflammation and protease activation, and strategies for prevention of inflammation-induced* *matrix degradation - a review*. International Journal of Cosmetic Science, 27(1), 17-34. https://doi.org/10.1111/j.1467-2494.2004.00241.x

Romanucci, V., D'Alonzo, D., Guaragna, A., Di Marino, C., Davinelli, S., Scapagnini, G., Di Fabio, G., & Zarrelli, A. **(2016)**. *Bioactive compounds of Aristotelia chilensis Stuntz and their pharmacological effects*. Current Pharmaceutical Biotechnology, 17(6), 513-523. https://doi.org/10.2174/1389201017666160114095246

Scanlon, V. C., & Sanders, T. **(2018)**. *essentials of anatomy and physiology*. F.A. Davis.

Schueller, R., & Romanowski, P. **(2016)**. *Multifunctional cosmetics*. CRC Press.

Wickett, R. R., & Visscher, M. O. **(2006)**. *Structure and function of the epidermal barrier*. American Journal of Infection Control, 34(10), S98-S110. https://doi.org/10.1016/j.ajic.2006.05.295

Winston, D., & Maimes, S. **(2007)**. *Adaptogens: Herbs for strength, stamina, and stress relief*. Inner Traditions / Bear & Co.

Yance, D. R. **(2013)**. *Adaptogens in medical herbalism: Elite herbs and natural compounds for mastering stress, aging, and chronic disease*. Simon & Schuster.

Yarnell, E. **(2003)**. *Phytochemistry and pharmacy for practitioners of botanical medicine*.

Zúñiga, G. E., Tapia, A., Arenas, A., Contreras, R. A., & Zúñiga-Libano, G. **(2017)**. *Phytochemistry and biological properties of Aristotelia chilensis a Chilean BlackBerry: A review*. Phytochemistry Reviews, 16(5), 1081-1094. https://doi.org/10.1007/s11101-017-9533-1

www.ingramcontent.com/pod-product-compliance
Lightning Source LLC
Chambersburg PA
CBHW040218220526
45473CB00001B/37